Sexuality and Disabilities: A Guide for Human Service Practitioners

Sexuality and Disabilities: A Guide for Human Service Practitioners

Romel W Mackelprang
Deborah Valentine
Editors

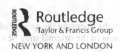

Routledge
Taylor & Francis Group
NEW YORK AND LONDON

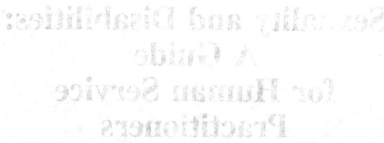

First Published by

The Haworth Press, Inc., 10 Alice Street, Binghamton, NY 13904-1580 USA

Transferred to Digital Printing 2010 by Routledge
270 Madison Ave, New York NY 10016
2 Park Square, Milton Park, Abingdon, Oxon, OX14 4RN

Sexuality and Disabilities: A Guide for Human Service Practitioners has also been published as *Journal of Social Work & Human Sexuality,* Volume 8, Number 2 1993.

Paperback edition published in 1996.

Cover design by Monica Seifert

Library of Congress Cataloging-in-Publication Data

Sexuality and disabilities : a guide for human service practitioners / Romel W. Mackelprang, Deborah Valentine, editors.
    p. cm.
    Includes bibliographical references.
    ISBN 0-7890-0092-X (alk. paper) ISBN: 1-56024-375-9 (alk. paper)
    1. Handicapped–United States–Sexual behavior. 2. Social work with the handicapped–United States. I. Mackelprang, Romel W, 1955- . II. Valentine, Deborah.
HQ30.5.S23 1993
306.7'087–dc20   93-354
                                                  CIP

Publisher's Note
The publisher has gone to great lengths to ensure the quality of this reprint but points out that some imperfections in the original may be apparent.

Dedication

To my supportive and loving family — Gene, Jason and Kesna Wells. And to the individuals and families involved in the rewards and struggles of developing and maintaining intimate relationships.

Deborah Valutine

My appreciation goes to Susan and our children, Rachel, Romel, Emily and Rebecca, for their love and support and to my parents who have always encouraged a thirst for understanding. Special thanks go to my clients and friends with disabilities from whom I have learned so much.

Romel W Mackelprang

Sexuality and Disabilities: A Guide for Human Service Practitioners

CONTENTS

ABOUT THE EDITORS

Romel W Mackelprang, MSW, DSW, is Assistant Professor at Eastern Washington University, School of Social Work and Human Services, Cheney and Spokane. He has published and produced educational materials on sexuality and disability. He has also researched and published on the topics of physical and neurological disabilities, health care policy and practice, and HIV/AIDS. He is currently directing a research project on disability and social work education, investigating issues such as curriculum, accessibility and faculty and student recruitment and retention.

Deborah Valentine, MSSW, PhD, is Associate Professor at the University of South Carolina, College of Social Work in Columbia. She has published on issues of child maltreatment, family violence, infertility, adoption, developmental disabilities, natural helping, and family relations. She has recently completed a research project investigating the psychosocial impact of assistance dog ownership for people with mobility or hearing impairments and another on policies of sexual harassment in the academic setting. Dr. Valentine is the Director of the Doctoral Program at the College of Social Work, University of South Carolina. She recently returned from a year sabbatical in Quito, Ecuador where she actively participated in a social action organization to address the needs of women and children.

Contributors

Pasquale J. Accardo, MD, is Professor of Pediatrics at St. Louis University. In that capacity, he serves as Director of the Division of Developmental Pediatrics and as Director of Ambulatory Pediatrics. His interest in the ability of adults with mental retardation to parent extends to his early years at the Kennedy Institute in Baltimore. Dr. Accardo has co-authored several textbooks in Developmental Pediatrics, and together with Dr. Whitman, co-authored the book *When a Parent is Mentally Retarded.*

Arlene Bowers Andrews, PhD, LISW, Associate Professor, College of Social Work, University of South Carolina, has worked in the victimization field for 15 years as an administrator and educator. Her primary interests are the development of community services systems for survivors and primary prevention of family problems. She is the author of *Victimization and Survivor Services* and several articles and training manuals.

Pamela S. Boyle, MS, has worked in the field of sexuality and disability for 16 years since receiving her Master's degree in Rehabilitation Counseling from Boston University. For eight and one half years, she was Coordinator of the Reproductive Health Care and Disability Program at Planned Parenthood of New York City. She is Past President of The Coalition on Sexuality and Disability and was the 1991 recipient of its Anne H. Berkman Memorial Service Award. An AASECT Certified Sex Counselor and Fellow of the American Board of Sexology, she now works full-time as a sexuality and disability consultant for several major habilitation and rehabilitation facilities in the New York City metropolitan area.

Romel W Mackelprang, MSW, DSW, is Assistant Professor, Inland Empire School of Social Work and Human Services, Eastern Washington University, Cheney, Washington.

xiii

Rita Rhodes, ACSW, PhD, is Assistant Professor at the University of South Carolina, College of Social Work in Columbia. She has published on issues of women and children and has a special interest in social welfare history.

Carol Sandowski, LCSW, ACSW, began her work with persons having physical disabilities while completing her MSW studies at Jane Addams Graduate School of Social Work, from which she graduated in 1975. Having several years of full time experience in physical rehabilitation, she has also worked in hospice, home health and Planned Parenthood. A licensed clinical social worker in Illinois, Mrs. Sandowski is an American Association of Sex Educators Counselors and Psychotherapists (AASECT) certified sex counselor. Mrs. Sandowski has numerous publications, including her book, *Sexuality Concerns When Illness or Disability Strikes,* published in 1989.

Gary R. Sigler, EdD, is Associate Professor of Applied Psychology at Eastern Washington University. His professional activities focus on issues concerning disability and the improvement of the social climate for individuals with disability. He has been a special education teacher, community college learning center instructor, paraprofessional trainer, and university professor in the area of exceptionality. His professional affiliations have included Council for Exceptional Children, National Rehabilitation Association, and American Association on Mental Deficiency.

Deborah Valentine, MSW, PhD, is Associate Professor, College of Social Work, University of South Carolina.

Lois Veronen, PhD, is Associate Professor of Psychology at Winthrop University. She is an early sexual assault researcher and spent ten years at the Crime Victim's Research and Treatment Center at the Medical University of South Carolina in Charleston, South Carolina before joining Winthrop's faculty. As director of a Victims of Crime Act project and Coordinator of Clinical Services of the South Carolina University Affiliated Program during 1989-1991 at Winthrop she identified and treated persons with developmental disabilities who have been victims of crime. She also has a private practice specializing in victims of violence and is a frequent expert witness in cases of battered women and rape victims in criminal and civil court.

Barbara Y. Whitman, PhD, is Associate Professor of Pediatrics at St. Louis University with additional teaching responsibilities at the School of Social Services. Trained as a family therapist, she has long been interested in families with special needs. In addition to the book co-authored with Dr. Accardo, Dr. Whitman together with Dr. Accardo and Dr. Tom Blondis have also recently published a book entitled *Attention Deficit Disorder and Hyperactivity in Children*. A third book, *A Dictionary of Developmental Disabilities* is in press.

Foreword

Although it has been unusual to discuss issues of sexuality and intimacy in relation to people with disabilities, the need for such discussions is becoming increasingly obvious. Social workers and other practitioners working with survivors of sexual assault and both adult and child protective services workers are becoming more aware of the need to identify, acknowledge and meet the particular needs of people with disabilities. Trends toward independent living and mainstreaming also call to our attention the needs of all human beings for intimacy. People with disabilities are speaking out more often and more loudly than ever before–demanding rights and the responsibilities that accompany education, marriage, parenthood and the full range of options afforded people without disabilities. Books such as *With Wings: An Anthology of Literature by and About Women with Disabilities* edited by Marsha Saxton and Florence Howe (1987), *With the Power of Each Breath: A Disabled Women's Anthology* edited by Susan E. Brown, Debra Connors and Nanci Stern (1985), and *Sexuality and Disability: Personal Perspectives* edited by David Bullard and Susan Knight (1982), are three such examples of this public and private wakening.

This volume, *Sexuality and Disabilities: A Guide for Human Service Practitioners* is a collection of eight articles selected to provide practitioners with an increased awareness and knowledge of the importance of providing services and the value of providing opportunities for people with disabilities. Three editorial decisions were made. First, the editors deliberately did not restrict discussions to a particular type or cluster of disabilities. The reader will find discussions that pertain to a wide range of disabilities including physical disabilities, developmental disabilities, mental retardation, learning disabilities and conditions which may have an impact on people later in life such as strokes, heart disease, or other chronic illnesses. It is the editors' intent to provide a broad brush approach to the topic–to provide an awareness that all people need individualized consideration and that the special needs of all individuals are important. Secondly, in seeking contributors, the editors sought out several authors who are "in the trenches"; that is, they are practitioners who have extensive experience in sexuality and disability. By including practitioners, the editors intend to give readers access to their knowledge, developed from the authors' years of practical expertise. Third, the editors chose not to limit discussions to issues of sexuality alone. Issues of sexuality are expanded to include issues of intimacy which are by definition intrinsic and essential. Thus, the articles in this volume include discussions of self-worth and identity as well as discussions which place sexuality in interpersonal contexts and networks of supportive relationships. Articles found in this volume include discussions of physical performance, the impact of disability on emotional relationships between partners, as well as the sources of support provided by neighbors, teachers or friends. Therefore, it is with the broadest of brush strokes that this volume on sexuality, intimacy and disabilities is offered to its readers.

The lead article, "Mental Retardation and Sexual Expression: An Historical Perspective," by Rita Rhodes provides the social and historical context by which current attitudes about sexuality, marriage and reproduction can be evaluated. Although there have been shifts in the position that persons with mental retardation should not form and maintain intimate relationships, attitudes change slowly and the kinds of support that are necessary for individuals and families to learn about partnerships and parenting are frequently not available for individuals and families with special needs.

The next four articles deal with the important topics of providing information, support and acknowledgement of issues of sexuality and intimacy to individuals in medical, educational or social service settings. Carol Sandowski explores attitudes of professionals in her article entitled "Responding to the Sexual Concerns of Persons with Disabilities." She concludes that most professionals are reluctant to talk about sex with patients and describes ways that hospital staff can be sensitized and trained to provide support for expressing sexuality to people with disabilities. In her article, "Training in Sexuality and Disability: Preparing Social Workers to Provide Services to Individuals with Disabilities," Pamela Boyle concurs that hospital staff are often educationally unprepared to address issues of intimacy and sexuality with people with disabilities and describes three components of a staff training program on sexuality and disability that can be implemented in habilitation, rehabilitation and hospital settings. Romel Mackelprang's article entitled "A Holistic Social Work Approach to Providing Sexuality Education and Counseling for Persons with Severe Disabilities" provides some very specific and helpful recommendations for sexuality education and counseling with people with spinal cord injuries and other acquired severe neurological disabilities. This article describes a model for meeting educational and counseling needs and to help people develop positive self-images and satisfying sexual lives. The attention that Dr. Mackelprang gives to able-bodied partners of individuals with severe disabilities is sensitively undertaken, reflects his wealth of knowledge in this area, and is a welcome addition to the literature. Gary Sigler and Romel Mackelprang urge professionals to consider the special needs of an additional group of individuals in the article "Cognitive Impairments: Psychosocial and Sexual Implications and Strategies for Social Work Intervention." They identify the special learning needs of people with cognitive impairments and suggest specific ways that educational programming, social work intervention and policy efforts can address these special needs.

The desires and needs of people to maintain healthy family relationships and supportive connections with others outside the family are the topics of the next three articles. Deborah Valentine describes the sources of support and stress of twenty-five families caring for children with developmental disabilities and argues that environmental stresses and social supports of parents of children with disabilities are important components of maintaining satisfying relationships. Dr. Valentine's research is especially valuable because it highlights the importance of extended families, communities and other formal and informal supports. Family functioning and intimacy are enhanced not only through clinical interventions, but through non-direct, community interventions that enhance family support. Barbara Whitman and Pasquale Accardo discuss a most important topic in their article "The Parent with Mental Retardation: Rights,

Responsibilities and Issues." After reviewing legal and ethical issues, the authors describe a model program serving parents with mental retardation and their children. The discussion is sensitively and knowledgeably presented and in addition to recommendations, challenges readers to struggle with several questions and concerns that are left unanswered and unresolved.

In the final article, Arlene Andrews and Lois Veronen provide an excellent discussion of vulnerabilities for sexual victimization in "Sexual Assault and People with Disabilities." After reviewing the literature and concluding that sexual assault is at least as common an occurrence for people with disabilities as for other people, the authors provide an analysis of special vulnerabilities and challenges that confront people with disabilities as they relate to sexual victimization. In addition, the authors offer specific recommendations to professionals for the design of prevention programs and victim assistance programs that are sensitive to the needs of all people, including those with special needs.

This book is intended to provide the reader with a better understanding of the issues of sexuality, intimacy and disabilities and offer suggestions for meeting needs that have been long ignored or stifled. As one person with a disability, acquired in his early 20s, stated, "When I was rehabilitated, they taught me how to dress, use a wheelchair, and even go to the bathroom again, but they ignored the important things in my life. I was taught all about survival, but nothing about living." It is the hope of the editors that this book will aid social workers in helping their clients get on with the process of "living."

Deborah Valentine
Romel Mackelprang

Mental Retardation
and Sexual Expression:
An Historical Perspective

Rita Rhodes

SUMMARY. This paper will examine the history of mental retardation within three distinct periods: the pre-Civil War, the turn-of-the-century and the 1960s. In each of these periods, professional and societal perceptions of mental retardation underwent significant revision. Despite changing perceptions, however, the constant feature in the treatment of individuals with mental retardation is society's resistance or denial of a sexual life for them. This paper will argue that the persistence of this factor in American society continues to present special challenges to advocates for individuals with mental retardation. Implications for social work practice are discussed.

Not unlike other minorities, the experiences permitted persons with mental retardation have been defined by the larger society. For this reason, any investigation into the sexual experience of individuals with mental retardation must take into account changing perceptions by the majority community. In addition, it will be argued that earlier societal views continue to inform what is considered acceptable sexual experience by the citizen with mental retardation.

Societal perceptions of individuals with mental retardation have varied over time. When perceived as harmless, the treatment accorded them could range from tolerance, indifference, amusement or special considerations as the "innocents of God." When viewed as a threat to the good of the community, however, treatment could extend from persecution to segregation in institutions such as prisons, poorhouses or hospitals. This paper will examine the history of mental retardation within three distinct transitional periods: the pre-Civil War, the turn-of-the-century and the 1960s. In each of these periods, professional and societal perceptions of mental retardation underwent significant revision. Despite changing perceptions, however, the constant feature in the treatment of individuals with mental retardation is society's resistance or denial of a sexual life for them.

NINETEENTH-CENTURY AMERICA

Mainstream Beliefs

In nineteenth-century America, individuals with mental retardation were not regarded as dangerous but more a nuisance factor in a society which valued individualism and competition. Society was largely indifferent to their condition except insofar as public assistance was required for their support. For those without resources, the almshouse became the last resort for persons with mental retardation and for other vulnerable populations. After describing conditions in one almshouse in 1838 in which "two married men and their wives, and one aged colored woman, two male idiots, a very old man, and eleven children" occupied one room with ten beds, the institutional officials reported their frustrations to the New York legislature: "the law compelled us to receive them [the insane and feebleminded], but neither the law nor any authority under it provided us the place to keep them in a proper manner" (Deutsch, 1949, p. 130). The plight of similar inhabitants was described by Dorothea Dix in her crusade to ameliorate the conditions of persons with mental illness and retardation that they encountered in jails and almshouses. Her immediate attention, however, was directed at providing asylums for those with mental illness.

Antebellum Reforms

Others, however, began to take an interest in the conditions of individuals with mental retardation. The origin of this attentiveness came from France. Edourd Seguin opened the first school for children with mental retardation in Paris in 1838. He interpreted "idiocy" as arrested development and set about developing educational methods to counter mental disabilities through the development of the body and training of the senses. French methods as well as the optimism they generated crossed the Atlantic, and a movement was begun in the United States to serve the educational needs of citizens with mental retardation. The timing for such efforts was propitious as antebellum America was an environment where social problems were thought surmountable by moral fervor and philanthropy. The expression of these latter was the founding of seven public training schools for children with mental retardation between 1848-1865.

American reformers believed that their interventions were best confined to work with children. An article published in the *American Journal of Education* in 1856 described their reasoning:

> In the countries where cretinism prevails, pupils over seven years are not considered as capable of successful instruction, but in other countries idiots are received up to the age of fifteen or sixteen, and in the English schools up to twenty-five or thirty, even. There is, however, far less hope of material progress in adults than in children—and it is hardly desirable that those beyond fourteen or fifteen should be placed under instruction. (Brockett, 1976, p. 81)

The purpose of instruction was to return these children to the community where they would hopefully support themselves. Even if unsuccessful in that endeavor, however, the moral training that children received would eradicate "bad and vicious habits" (Pim, 1976, p. 100).

One of the "vicious habits" that was of most concern to reformers was "self-abuse" or masturbation. Masturbation was thought to violate "natural law" and so contribute to the growth of mental retardation both in its performers and in their progeny. In his report to the Massachusetts Legislature in 1848, Samuel Howe, superintendent of the first training school for citizens with mental retardation, noted that ten cases of the "idiocy of the children" could be "manifestly attributable to this sin of the parent" (Howe, 1976,

p. 56). For other "self-abusers," the consequences could be exhibited in their own lives:

> There are among those enumerated in this report some who not long ago were considered young gentlemen and ladies, but who are now moping idiots,–idiots of the lowest kind; lost to all reason, to all moral sense, to all shame,–idiots who have but one thought, one wish, one passion,–and that is, the further indulgence in the habit which has loosed the silver cord even in their early youth, which has already wasted, and, as it were, dissolved, the fibrous part of their bodies, and utterly extinguished their minds. (Howe, 1976, p. 54)

Convinced of the etiology of "idiocy," professionals who worked with these children took pains to ensure that their clients would undergo no further mental decline because of their sexual habits. Howe was pleased to note that in his experience:

> There is one remarkable and valuable fact to be learned respecting this vice, from observation of idiots, and that is, that some of them, though they have no idea of right and wrong, no sense of shame, and no moral restraint, are nevertheless entirely free from it. They could never have been in the practice of it, else they never would have abandoned it. (Howe, 1976, p. 56)

Howe further concluded that "it is handed from one to another like contagion; and that those who are not exposed to the contagion are not likely to contact the dreadful habit of it" (Howe, 1976, p. 57). With an understanding of masturbation as both contagious and habit-forming, Howe recommended vigilance as the primary method of dealing with sexual explorations. Howe made the same recommendations for the parents of children with and without disabilities: "It behooves every parent, especially those whose children (of either sex) are obliged to board and sleep with other children . . . to have a constant and watchful eye over them, with a view to this insidious and pernicious habit. The symptoms of it are easily learned, and, if once seen, should be immediately noticed" (Howe, 1976, p. 55). Howe and his contemporaries did not differ from other educators in both their warnings and their vigilance against sexual activity among their charges.

1870-1890

Transition

While the generation of professionals who confined their work to children was still in the field, the emergence of others emphasized the needs of adult clients who were considered inappropriate for lives in the community. The professional literature of the period suggested that institutional life would not only better accommodate the needs of these adults but also successfully shelter them from the dangers of the larger community. The president of the American Association on Mental Deficiency (AAMD), A. C. Rogers, emphasized at the annual meeting in 1890 "the necessity of retaining our pupils and wards for life, not as prisoners, but as pupils, patients, members of a great family living a life of usefulness amid cheerful and happy surroundings" (Sloan & Stevens, 1976, p. 19).

In response to this change in institutional direction, was a corresponding change in the perception and treatment of clients. Inhabitants were increasingly perceived as needing care and protection rather than training and education. At the AAMD in 1890, Rogers summarized the declining expectations: "Once feebleminded, always feebleminded, only in a less degree" (Sloan & Stevens, 1976, p. 19). Reflecting the professional paternalism that came to predominate, Isaac N. Kerlin, superintendent of the Pennsylvania Training School, articulated his vision for the future in a report to the National Conference on Charities and Corrections in 1885:

. . . here and there scattered over the country, may be 'villages of the simple,' made up of the warped, twisted, and incorrigible, happily contributing to their own and the support of those more lowly,—'cities of refuge,' in truth; havens in which all shall live contentedly, because no longer misunderstood nor taxed with exactions beyond their mental or moral capacity. They 'shall go out no more,' and 'they shall neither marry nor be given in marriage,' in those havens dedicated to incompetency. (White and Wolfensberger, 1969, p. 7)

Implicit in this view was an understanding that a sexual life that might enlarge this population was not to be encouraged.

Social Darwinism and the Eugenic Movement

Interspersed with the ideas on the need for protection of persons with mental retardation was an increasingly articulated concern about the danger that such individuals represented to society itself. This latter perception was shaped by an intellectual climate that sought a social application for the concepts of evolution and natural selection that had been described in Charles Darwin's *Origin of the Species*. Francis Galton, a cousin of Darwin's, used the term "eugenics" (from the Greek for "well-born") in 1883 to describe "the study of the agencies under social control that may improve or impair the racial qualities of future generations either physically or mentally" (Deutsch, 1949, p. 358). The movement emphasized the dominance of heredity and sought to encourage the reproduction of socially desirable individuals (positive eugenics) and discourage the reproduction of the undesirable (negative eugenics).

The hereditary transmission of social problems was an ideal way for both professionals and the general public to understand the changing and often frightening environment of industrial America. Numbers of "scientific" genealogical works were produced which demonstrated the social effects of "degenerate" families over time. The most influential of these was a reported history of the Kallikak Family published in 1912 by Henry H. Goddard, director of the research laboratory at the Vineland Training School in New Jersey, which traced the descendants of the great-great grandmother of one of the patients at Vineland. Goddard concluded that of 480 descendants, 143 were persons with mental retardation. Importantly, almost three quarters of the descendants were judged to be "degenerates" of one kind or other (Farber, 1968, p. 31).

The most telling of these genealogical works, however, was that of the Jukes Family originally published by Richard L. Dugdale in 1877. Dugdale traced the criminal activities of the Jukes family and concluded that bad environmental conditions produced such behavior in generations of family members. In 1915, however, Arthur H. Estabrook re-examined Dugdale's original work and concluded in a re-published study of the family that one half of the Jukes were individuals with mental retardation and that all the criminal members of the family were. According to one student of the period, "what was regarded in 1877 as primarily a problem in criminal degeneracy, became in 1915, mainly a problem of mental deficiency" (Rosen, Clark, & Kivitz, 1976, pp. 145-6).

These works contributed to the public and professional belief that mental retardation was both inherited and associated with social problems. Demographic evidence was gathered to bolster both of these beliefs. The federal census in its 1890 report disclosed that persons with mental retardation were more likely to have insane or "feebleminded" relatives than either the deaf or the blind. Other studies were produced that "proved" that a large proportion of prisoners, alcoholics and prostitutes were "mentally retarded" (Farber, 1968, p. 27). Together, the impression upon professionals and the general public was that the larger community needed to be protected from a menacing and dangerous population. Walter E. Fernald, superintendent of the Massachusetts School for the Feeble-Minded, warned his colleagues at the 1912 AAMD annual meeting: "It has been truly said that feeblemindedness is the mother of crime, pauperism and degeneracy. It is certain that the feebleminded and the progeny of the feebleminded constitute one of the great social and economic burdens of modern times" (Sloan & Stevens, 1976, p. 76). For professionals as well as the general public, this population had become "the most potent, if not the sole, source of all social evils" (Vecoli, 1960, p. 191).

Given the overwhelming "scientific" evidence of the period that nominated mental retardation as a source of a plethora of social problems, those who had concerned themselves with such problems were left with an unsure role. The National Conference of Charities and Corrections struggled with the issue beginning in the 1890s and eventually advocated prevention as the significant role for its members. The keynote address of the 1915 meeting, for example, featured Marvin Barr, of the Pennsylvania Training School at Elwyn, who declared "that the prevention of the transmission of mental defect is the paramount duty of the hour" (Deutsch, 1949, p. 361). Edward T. Devine of the New York Charity Organization Society, also advised that "there is much of this eugenics program with which social workers may sympathize and in which they should clearly cooperate. The permanent segregation, during the reproductive years of life, of the feeble-minded, the insane, the incorrigibly criminal, and the hopelessly ineffective . . . would enormously reduce the total social burden" (Devine, 1912, pp. 44-45).

1890-1920

Institutional Segregation

Public and professional perception alike were increasingly likely to view individuals with mental retardation as a dangerous class from whom society needed protection. Segregation was the first eugenic measure to win widespread support. Professionals, unlike their predecessors, regularly advocated for the permanent institutionalization of those with mild forms of mental retardation. In an address to the AAMD in 1902, Martin Barr described the professional consensus: "Without formal expression emanating from our association as a body there is yet, I believe, a consensus that abandons the hope long cherished of a return of the imbecile to the world" (Barr, 1976, p. 101). With the victory of this viewpoint, training schools were converted to custodial institutions while other institutions were enlarged or created. The numbers of institutionalized reflected this new mandate and institutionalized individuals with mental retardation increased from 14,000 in 1910 to nearly 43,000 in 1923 (Rosen, Clark & Kivitz, 1976, p. 146). The possibility of a segregated solution appealed to an editorialist in the *Journal of Psycho-Asthenics*, the official publication of the AAMD, in 1899:

> If the day ever comes–let us say bravely when the day comes– that all or nearly all, the degenerates are gathered into industrial, celibate communities, how rapidly the 'White Man's Burden' of distress, pauperism, and disease, which he must be taxed to support, begins to diminish. (Tyor & Bell, 1984, p. 104)

According to this vision, a segregated, celibate population of the mentally retarded was a viable solution to the social problems of turn-of-the-century America.

Institutional Life

The professionals who were charged with the care of this "dangerous" minority took their responsibility seriously. Within institutional life itself, the sexes were segregated to prevent any occasion for sexual activity. In a 1902 address to the AAMD, Martin Barr advised on the experiences of his institution:

> The separation of the sexes is another problem which experience is slowly defining. At Elwyn teachers are a unit in declaring there is nothing gained in co-education, even in convenience, while nerve strain in disciplining is greatly increased, and a re-arrangement of classes according to sex rather than grade is already deemed advisable. (Barr, 1976, p. 103)

Given the increased demand on the facilities by adults who would not be discharged to the community, administrators responded by the development of a colony system. Several state institutions who had struggled with the issue of space had purchased farm land for the establishment of colonies. These would be inhabited by adults who had completed their training but would not be eligible for parole into the community. Unlike the early training schools, rural areas were considered ideal for these "colonists." Walter A. Fernald described the first farm colony in 1902: "We have created a little community suited to the need and capacity of these feeble-minded boys, or men—a little world made for them, where they live the natural life of a country boy" (Tyor and Bell, 1984, p. 87). Once safely ensconced in institutions, persons with mental retardation could leave behind the label of dangerous in favor of the child-like image favored by their caretakers.

Marriage Restriction

Another eugenic method, the restriction of marriages, was obviously for a non-institutionalized population and so did not receive the whole-hearted support of the eugenicists and professionals who believed that the proper place of individuals with mental retardation was within institutions. The question of practicality was a concern in that there was usually not a mechanism in place to deter anyone from obtaining a marriage license. The practicality factor was critical for eugenicists who argued that "it would be as sensible to hope to control by legislation, the mating of rabbits" (Tyor and Bell, 1984, p. 119). Goddard also dismissed the attempt at marriage restriction: "It may be that we shall be willing to sterilize all of the borderline cases and then there will be no longer any objection to their marrying" (Tyor and Bell, 1984, p. 119).

Sterilization

Sterilization, unlike restricted marriage, was at first considered a procedure that would be used in conjunction with institutionalized individuals with mental retardation. Marvin Barr was a leading advocate of sterilization who recommended the procedure for both institutional as well as eugenic purposes. In 1902, Barr in his office as Chief Physician of The Pennsylvania Training School, delineated the benefits of sterilization for the institutionalized:

. . . the whole matter might be simplified and the nervous atmosphere relieved by early invoking the aid of surgical interference to secure at once safety to society, less tension to community life, and greater liberty, therefore greater happiness, to the individual. This has taken distinct form in an effort on the part of several members of my own Board (whom I accompanied to Harrisburg last winter) to seek legislative authorization for the asexualization upon admission to institutions of those adjudged mentally and morally defective. The bill, which passed both houses, was finally lost through the timidity of the Governor. (Barr, 1976, pp. 103-4)

Others were not so sure and worried about the possible violation of individual rights. The National Conference of Corrections and Charities, for one, had majority and minority reports read at its meeting in 1903, the majority supporting segregation but not sterilization. The minority view was presented by Mary E. Perry, Vice President of the Missouri State Board of Charities and Corrections, who argued her support of sterilization in the context of child welfare: "It is time we looked this question squarely in the face and as it is humane, so it is righteous if resorted to for the sake of the child" (Tyor and Bell, 1984, p. 103). Edward Devine (1912) in his text *The Family and Social Work* opposed sterilization as "a policy of very doubtful expediency" (p. 46). Social workers continued to have difficulty seeking a consensus on the issue and one worker in New York complained that the state sterilization law "was neither proposed nor urged, . . . by those who have been prominently concerned with social work in this state. . . . Neither was it opposed" (Tyor and Bell, 1984, pp. 119-120). E. A. Ross, a professor and Progressive, however, had no such difficulty in expressing his opinion: "Sterilization is not nearly so terrible as hanging a man, and the chances of sterilizing the fit are not nearly so great as are the chances of hanging the innocent" (Vecoli, 1960, p. 196).

Despite Barr's best efforts, Indiana rather than Pennsylvania became the first state to pass a sterilization law in 1907 and by 1917, fourteen other states permitted the operation (Tyor and Bell, 1984, p. 118). Indiana's statute permitted the sterilization of "confirmed criminals, idiots, imbeciles and rapists" (Deutsch, 1949, p. 370). An important feature of the Indiana statute was that the sterilization would proceed when judged "that procreation was inadvisable and that there was no probability of the subject's mental improvement" (Deutsch, 1949, p. 370). Both of these criteria were the usual beliefs about their clients held by those who worked in the field of mental retardation. In other states, candidates for sterilization were usually evaluated by boards of professionals who were charged to judge as to whether an individual was "hereditarily feeble-minded." By 1921, 3,233 sterilizations had been performed on individuals with mental retardation and other classes who met the criteria (Tyor and Bell, 1984, p. 119).

Women: A Separate Case

The concern about women with mental retardation became something of an obsession among administrators and legislators by the turn-of-the-century (Scheerenberger, 1983, p. 124). This concern was not limited to professionals in the field of mental retardation. The Philadelphia Department of Public Health and Charity warned in a 1910 pamphlet that "practically all poor feeble-minded women at large become mothers of illegitimate children soon after reaching the age of puberty" (Tyor and Bell, 1984, p. 117). For those with an eugenic orientation, women with mental retardation were considered not only to be sexually promiscuous but to enjoy a higher fertility rate than their "normal" sisters. In a paper entitled "The Burden of Feeblemindedness" presented at the 1912 meeting of the AAMD, Walter E. Fernald described the behavior of women with mental retardation: "Feebleminded women are almost invariably immoral and if at large, usually become carriers of venereal disease or give birth to children who are as defective as themselves. The feebleminded woman who marries is twice as prolific as the normal woman" (Sloan and Stevens, 1976, p. 76).

The notion that women could be sexual was a disagreeable one to many professionals whose idea of a proper woman excluded sexual desire. For some, the identification of mental retardation itself could be assumed by the presence of female sexual activity outside of marriage. In New York, the trustees of the New York State Custodial Asylum for Feeble-Minded Women saw their purpose as caring for women who because of mental defect are "ungoverned and easily yielding to lust" (Tyor, 1977, p. 480). In Massachusetts, a board of trustees struggled with whether "inordinate sexual passion on the part of a young woman [is] to be regarded by the trustees as sufficient evidence of feeble-mindedness to hold her as an inmate of this institution" (Tyor, 1977, p. 481). Women were often admitted or retained in custodial institutions for reasons that had more to do with the sexual expectations of those who evaluated them than it did their own mental deficits.

Institutions responded to the sexual threat that women represented by increasing efforts to admit and retain adult women. Indiana, for instance, extended the female age limit for admission from 16 to 45 in 1901. The law also provided for permanent custodial care for "all feebleminded female imbeciles in the state under the childbearing age" (Sloan and Stevens, 1976, p. 51). By 1919, institutions solely for women existed in New York, New Jersey and

Pennsylvania (Scheerenberger, 1983, p. 159). Women with mild retardation (the high-grade female "imbecile") were considered the most dangerous by Walter Fernald:

> They are certain to become sexual offenders and to spread venereal disease or to give birth to degenerate children. Their numerous progeny usually become public charges as diseased or neglected children, imbeciles, epileptics, juvenile delinquents or later on as adult paupers or criminals. The segregation of this class should be rapidly extended until all not adequately guarded at home are placed under strict sexual quarantine. Hundreds of known cases of this sort are now at large because the institutions are overcrowded. (Sloan and Stevens, 1976, pp. 76-77)

1920-1950

Continuity and Change

By the 1920s, the heyday of the eugenics movement had passed and professionals were re-examining their own eugenics orientation. As early as 1918 even Walter Fernald, an active superintendent who had been an early supporter of permanent segregation, could report:

> There are both bad feeble-minded and good feeble-minded, and . . . not all of the feeble-minded are criminalists and socialists and immoral and antisocial; we know they are not. We know that a lot of the feeble-minded are generous, faithful, and pure-minded. I never lose an opportunity to repeat what I am saying now, that we have really slandered the feeble-minded. Some of the sweetest and most beautiful characters I have ever known have been feeble-minded people. (Cegelka and Prehm, 1982, p. 60)

The perception had begun to shift to a more positive view point that regarded individuals with mental retardation as "pure-minded" and "sweetest." But whether as "dangerous" or "pure-minded," neither characterization was likely to accommodate their sexual needs. And although in decline, an eugenic orientation would remain a powerful perspective from which individuals with mental retardation would continue to be judged.

In addition to a changing perspective, numbers alone dictated that professionals needed to rethink the viability of permanent custodial care. Walter Fernald noted the increase in the identified population in 1913: "The field of mental defect has been so broadened and extended as to include large groups of persons who would not have been included even a decade ago. Naturally this extension has been almost entirely in the higher grades of defect" (Tyor and Bell, 1984, p. 111). In response to a changing perspective and the pressures of numbers, some administrators sought to shift the mission of their respective institutions away from permanent custodial care. The eugenic influence, however, remained powerful in decision-making about those who would be allowed to go on parole or those who would be returned as failures.

Professionals who were willing to experiment with the idea of parole, pointed to the existence of a gender differential in successful community placement. Howard W. Potter, who was director of research at Letchworth Village in New York, reported in 1926 that "males are far more successful in extra-institutional adaptation than are females" (Potter and McCollister, 1976, p. 136). Attempting to account for this differential, he reported that "the males were returned mainly on account of general incorrigibility and the girls principally for tendencies or actual expressions of sex delinquency" (Potter and McCollister, 1976, p. 140). Potter concluded that the eugenic considerations still prevailed in the institutional definition of success:

> Many of our paroles would have been considered as having made a satisfactory extra-institutional adjustment if we had disregarded what one might term a normal interest in the opposite sex. It should be emphasized that the patients we placed on parole but rarely indulged promiscuously in sex activities. They reacted to an instinctive urge for procreation which is resident in every living thing and the matter of eugenics has made us regard even the rather normal flirtations of our

patients with the opposite sex as a sufficient reason for cancelling their parole. In other words if we had put our "eugenical pride" in our pocket we would have had a far greater percentage of successes on parole. (Potter and McCollister, 1976, p. 141)

Selective Sterilization

The general reluctance to put their "eugenical pride in their pocket" forced institutional officials to reconsider their earlier position that "sterilization should be used in conjunction with segregation and not as a substitute for it" (Tyor and Bell, 1984, p. 119). Alexander Johnson who earlier had opposed sterilization in support of segregation, by 1916 favored it as "a real necessity" given "the impossibility of segregating all the morons" (Tyor and Bell, 1984, p. 119). In addition, institutional administrators no longer recommended sterilization as a broad-based intervention but came to support it as a selective procedure. Edgar A. Doll, president of the AAMD in 1936, addressed the association: "The legal and academic aspects of sterilization present difficulties of such moment, however, that compulsory sterilization cannot be viewed with much optimism, however great its practical value might be" (Sloan and Stevens, 1976, p. 159). Selective sterilization was considered most appropriate for individuals with mild mental retardation who would be candidates for a return to the community (Scheerenberger, 1983, p. 190).

The most ambitious program that linked sterilization and parole was that of Sonoma State Home in California where 4,310 residents underwent the surgery between 1919 and 1943. At Sonoma, sterilization was "a standard procedure for patients about to be paroled who are still in their reproductive period" (Scheerenberger, 1983, p. 226). For another institution, the failure to sterilize was held to contribute to the problems of paroled women:

Regarding sterilization, these girls who have gone out from our institution and have come back as failures would have been successes if they had been sterilized. . . . They are successes—they have good personalities, but from our standard and the standards of the social workers they are failures. They cannot go out year after year and keep absolutely straight. (Potter and McCollister, 1976, p. 143)

The support for sterilization was sanctioned by the 1927 U.S. Supreme Court decision *Buck v. Bell* which upheld the constitutionality of the Virginia sterilization statute. Justice Holmes delivered the opinion of the court:

> We have seen more than once that the public welfare may call upon the best citizens for their lives. It would be strange if it could not call upon those who already sap the strength of the State for these lesser sacrifices, often not felt to be such by those concerned, in order to prevent our being swamped with incompetence. It is better for all the world, if instead of waiting to execute degenerate offspring for crime, or to let them starve for their imbecility, society can prevent those who are manifestly unfit from continuing their kind. The principle that sustains compulsory vaccination is broad enough to cover the cutting of the Fallopian tubes. . . . Three generations of imbeciles are enough. (Macklin and Gaylin, 1981, p. 207)

This decision simplified the passage of other sterilization laws and by 1936, twenty-five states had such laws. All of the statutes included citizens with mental retardation among the groups subject to sterilization (Deutsch, 1949, pp. 370-71). The state statutes were a mixture of both compulsory and voluntary sterilizations. Voluntary sterilizations, however, included those performed solely with the consent of a legal guardian.

Despite legal sanctions and strong professional support in certain quarters for the sterilization of the "feebleminded," the policy was largely a failure. The vast majority of individuals with mental retardation, whether in the community or in institutions, did not undergo this procedure. From 1907 until January 1, 1946, 22,153 legal sterilizations were performed on persons categorized as "feebleminded." This represented a small percentage of the identified population. In addition, sterilization efforts were concentrated in areas where the eugenics movement was strong. Of the 45,127 sterilizations performed on all groups during this period, 17,835 were performed in California where the movement was particularly well-funded (Deutsch, 1949, p. 372). The eugenics movement, moreover, would be even more difficult to sustain after World War II when the atrocities performed upon vulnerable groups, including the mentally retarded, were publicized.

Institutional Life

Custodial care remained the primary purpose of institutions for persons with mental retardation and limited resources ensured that care was very minimal. In addition, the quality of institutional life further declined during the Depression and War years when institutions had to compete for shrinking government funds. The decline of familial resources, moreover, reduced the numbers discharged as well as increased the numbers admitted and thereby heightened the economic stress of institutions (Scheerenberger, 1983, p. 200). Between 1934 and 1943, the number of persons with mental retardation in institutions increased by 40 percent (Scheerenberger, 1983, p. 240). Overcrowding was a fact of institutional life and institutions with populations of 30% to 40% above bed capacity were not exceptional (Scheerenberger, 1983, p. 241).

A strict enforcement of policies regarding the segregation of the sexes was the usual institutional response to the pressure of numbers. In a discussion of co-educational versus single-sex facilities, however, most administrators favored the former as more representative of the outside world. Mary Wolf was an administrator who dissented from this view:

> I would like to challenge the statement that the life in a bi-sex institution is normal. This may be true while the inmates are children, but unfortunately children grow up, and just as soon as they reach a certain age, there are safeguards erected between the two sexes, so that practically the same situation exists as in a one-sex institution. Beyond a certain limit, connection between the two sexes cannot be permitted in a two-sex institution after the children are grown. (Scheerenberger, 1983, p. 197)

Institutional officials warned inmates against any contact with the opposite sex and sought to provide "strict supervision of activities" as a "curb upon the development of such relationships" (Abel & Kinder, 1942, p. 124). One young woman successfully incorporated institutional policy into her own philosophy of life: "Keep away from boys. That's what they say and what I say" (Abel & Kinder, 1942, p. 125).

POST WORLD WAR II

In the two decades immediately following the War, the living conditions of persons with mental retardation did not differ significantly from the pre-War years. The promise and prosperity of post-War America eluded those with mental retardation; the $5.57 per diem spent on the institutionalized in 1964 compared unfavorably with that spent on zoo animals (Scheerenberger, 1987, p. 224). The institutionalized population itself, moreover, continued to increase from 128,145 in 1950 to a peak of 193,188 in 1967 (Stroman, 1989, p. 130). But despite the direction that the numbers reflected, it was precisely during those years that the forces of change were being mobilized. The activism of parents' groups, the Civil Rights Movement, pro-active litigation, the election of John Kennedy, institutional exposes, and the increased self-criticism of professionals and institutional officials, led to the deinstitutionalization and normalization movements of the 1970s and 1980s.

The concepts of deinstitutionalization and normalization guided the efforts of both professionals and family members as they planned services for individuals with mental retardation. A policy of deinstitutionalization sought to reduce the population of institutions by both returning residents to the community and discouraging the admission of new clients. Consistent with this policy was the movement for normalization that supported the right of individuals with mental retardation to have access to "conditions of everyday life which are as close as possible to the norms and patterns of the mainstream of society" (Nirje, 1976, p. 363). Self-determination, in turn, is an implicit component of the principle of normalization. And for growing numbers of individuals with mental retardation, self-determination was manifested by a desire to develop social-sexual relationships that increasingly included marriage and parent-hood.

The desire for normalcy and intimacy made marriage prominent on the agenda of discharged clients from institutions. The work of Robert Edgerton (1967) indicated a high value placed on marriage by the discharged patients that he studied during the 1950s. A male participant in Edgerton's study stated:

> Before I was married I never used to have the same kind of life as other people. I was left out of so many things. Now that I got my wife (an ex-patient) I feel like I'm OK. I feel like I'm just as good as anybody. (p. 154)

Marriage for many individuals with mental retardation is a sign of self-esteem and independence and represents normalization more than any other undertaking. A journalist, in an account of the marriage of his brother and sister-in-law, reported his brother's request of the minister who was performing the ceremony: "Tell them (the wedding guests) that getting married is like coming out of retarda-tion" (Meyers, 1978, p. 100). And Edgerton (1967) concluded from his interviews with discharged residents who had subsequently mar-ried: "It would seem that the sexual and marital lives of these retarded persons are more 'normal' and better regulated than we could possibly have predicted from a knowledge of their pre-hospi-tal experiences and their manifest intellectual deficits" (p. 126). Other research suggests that the value placed on marriage by indi-viduals with mental retardation has led to long-lasting unions (Scheerenberger, 1987, p. 189).

With an extension of the Civil Rights Movement of the 1960s, the legal obstacles to marriage and parenthood for those individuals with mental retardation were either challenged in courts or let to remain on the books without actual enforcement. As of 1980, for example, 33 states still restricted the right of persons with mental retardation to marry. The reality, however, was that by 1960 these were not enforced and the courts rejected appeals to annul mar-riages on the basis of mental retardation (Scheerenberger, 1987, p. 188). By 1960, the actual practice of sterilization as well had become quite limited although 26 states still had laws that provided for the sterilization of persons with mental retardation (Scheerenberger, 1987, p. 189). In 1974, the U.S. Department of Health, Education, and Welfare issued regulations that offered safeguards to individuals regarding non-consensual sterilization contributing to a further decline in the practice (Scheerenberger, 1987, p. 192).

During the decades of the 1970s and 1980s, the thinking that had scrupulously guarded the rights of the larger society at the expense of citizens with mental retardation shifted to a position based almost exclusively on the protection of individual rights (Irvine, 1988; Melton & Scott, 1984). Even the support of parents for the sterilization of their child was not considered a secure protection of the best interests of the individual. The Supreme Court of Colorado in 1981 demonstrated the magnitude of the change:

> It is not the welfare of society, or the convenience or peace of
> mind of parents or guardians that these standards are intended
> to protect. The purpose of the standards is to protect the health
> of the minor retarded person, and to prevent that person's
> fundamental procreative rights from being abridged. (Scheer-
> enberger, 1987, p. 193)

Many states removed eugenic sterilization statutes but have not replaced them with legislation that would provide for voluntary sterilization under specific conditions (Passer, Rauh, Chamberlain, McGrath, & Burket, 1984). The ability to obtain a voluntary sterilization is also part of the normalization of sexuality and has been advocated as early as 1974 by the American Association on Mental Deficiency: "Since sterilization is a method of contraception available to most North American adults, this option should be open to most retarded citizens as well" (Scheerenberger, 1987, p. 192). The legal issue of voluntary sterilization and informed consent is complex and has yet to be resolved satisfactorily by the courts (Dickin & Ryan, 1983). The result is significant legal obstacles such that individuals with mental retardation can be "left in the quandary of having the courts protect their fundamental rights and not allow sterilization, yet not being able to exercise the fundamental right not to procreate" (Irvine, 1988, p. 110).

Beyond legal issues, another factor that intrudes upon the efforts of persons with mental retardation to "normalize" their sexual activity is the opposition of the larger society. In one 1970 opinion poll, 53.9% objected to persons with mental retardation marrying; in another taken the same year, 80% objected to persons with mental retardation dating those of normal intelligence (Scheerenberger, 1987, p. 189). A more significant impediment to sexual relationships, however, can be the opposition of family members themselves. While family members are often strong supporters of independent living consistent with the principle of normalization, they are more reluctant to approve a sexual life for their relatives. There is at least the suggestion in this resistance that one of the last aspects of normalization granted by the community is a sexual life for those labeled "mentally retarded."

Concern for parenting abilities of individuals is a major consideration for those who disapprove of sexual relationships for individuals with mental retardation (Heshusius, 1981). It has been argued, however, that a position of "normalization must include normal sexuality, including the right to bear children" (Edgerton, 1979, p. 97). The reality, moreover, is that the expectation of parenthood after marriage is a likelihood that is held by many couples with mental retardation (Heshusius, 1981; Monat, 1982). One groom, for example, stated his parenting intentions to his journalist brother: "That's what regular people do. They get married and have children and a house. That's what we wanted too" (Meyers, 1978, p. 107).

This determination to create a family is often alarming to parents and others involved with the couple who fear that the complexities of childrearing may overwhelm the couple and prove harmful to the child. The judgment of what constitutes adequate parenting is unclear as is the potential for successful parenting if these couples are the recipients of training and support. Parenting competency, while beyond the scope of this paper, is a complex issue that is not necessarily related to intelligence. Leo Kanner (1949) argued "that to a large extent independent of the IQ, fitness for parenthood is determined by emotional involvements and relationships" (p. 5). These qualities, however, are more difficult to measure than intelligence and the struggle to address competency in parenting behavior must "avoid setting a standard for minimally adequate parental care that is higher than the standard applied to nonretarded parents" (Melton & Scott, 1984, p. 42).

Despite ongoing legal and social problems that are not easily resolved, a sexual life for individuals with mental retardation is more feasible than in earlier periods. The removal of legal constraints upon the ability to marry as well as to procreate expanded the opportunities to secure a sexual life for those individuals with mental retardation. The freedom and ability to exercise sexual expression also received a positive formulation with the growing acceptance of the concept of normalization. As part of the normalization movement, not only did sexual prohibitions begin to be removed for persons with mental retardation but standards of behavior were created that increasingly expected participation in a full range of activities that included sexual expression. The principle of normalization is not static and has itself become a source of dispute and criticism. Nevertheless, as a positive concept it has served to expand the expectations of those involved in the field of mental retardation as well as to counter the stigmatization and stereotyping that is sustained by deeply-rooted societal values that continue to impede the sexual expression of individuals with mental retardation.

IMPLICATIONS FOR SOCIAL WORK

A survey of mental retardation in the United States in different historical periods illustrates the recurrence of certain themes around the topic of sexuality and mental retardation. The subject of heredity continues to be an issue which has the potential to inhibit sexual activity. The ongoing popularity of the work of Arthur Jensen and William Shockley suggests that eugenic arguments continue to shape the thinking of many Americans who believe in a linkage between social welfare and genes. Those who hold such opinions advocate that those with "defective" genes should not be allowed to perpetuate them. Advocacy and educational efforts must be extended to counteract the over-simplified understanding of human genetics and the role of inheritance in the causation of mental handicaps.

The historical record also suggests that society continues to conceptualize individuals with mental retardation as a homogeneous and undifferentiated population. This perception is at odds with the particularly American ideology of support for individual rights. The extension of these rights has been a slow and tedious process that has been haltingly applied to women, minorities and finally, individuals with handicaps. The ongoing fight and resistance to extend individual rights to persons with mental retardation suggests that the larger American society still retains perceptions that stigmatize this population as "child-like" or "dangerous" rather than a population as diverse as the "normal" population to whom it is unfavorably compared.

In order to support the individual with mental retardation as unique and capable of sexual intimacy, interventions must be designed that address the diversity of clients' needs around sexuality issues as they progress through the life cycle. Ongoing sex education is necessary as individuals sexually mature and move from roles as dependent children into more independent adult roles. The transition through adolescence is difficult for many and more so for those who do not have ready access to materials and companions who might be knowledgeable about sexual matters (David, Smith, & Friedman, 1976). Sex education courses with appropriate materials and teaching methods that match learning styles are critical for school-age individuals with mental retardation.

For adults, ongoing sexuality courses that include information on meeting psychosocial-sexual needs as well as current information on birth control options are pivotal. This training also should address the sexual behaviors and attitudes of the community in which adults reside so as to promote understanding as well as safety (Heshusius, 1981). Sex counseling groups are also recommended as an intervention for ongoing learning experiences as regards relationships, feelings and acceptable private and public behaviors (Dickerson, 1981; Monat, 1982). Counseling as to whether to pursue parenthood must be individualized and with such counseling, "most retarded women are able to be responsible for their own bodies and can decide whether or not they want to become pregnant" (Dickerson, 1981, p. 131). If parenthood becomes a choice, interventions are crucial as these individuals struggle to understand prenatal, birth and child development issues deprived of the educational experiences and materials available to their "normal" counterparts.

In addition, the apprehension about women with mental retardation continues to influence their treatment. The individual rights that are an issue for men are made more difficult for women who must labor under the double burden that comes from misperceptions about their handicap as well as their sex. Women with mental retardation still labor under the burden of being considered irresponsible about sex and unteachable about birth control and menstrual hygiene. The result is that women are more likely than men to be identified as candidates for involuntary sterilization although this procedure is now rare for those individuals considered "mildly retarded." The usual petitions for sterilization are based upon arguments that cite the need for contraception in the event that a woman is sexually abused or as a remedy for ongoing problems with menstrual hygiene (Melton & Scott, 1984). Alternatives might include interventions which address prevention of the sexual abuse itself rather than sterilization which does not prevent sexual abuse and, in fact, may actually increase its probability (Melton & Scott, 1984). In addition, training in mental hygiene and birth control might prove viable alternatives to sterilization although "the barrenness of the literature with respect to contraception training is almost matched by the state of research on menstrual-hygiene training" (Melton & Scott, 1984, pp. 42-43). While sterilization needs to remain an option, alternatives need to be considered to ensure a full range of options for women with mental retardation.

The needs of the individual with mental retardation are also supported by interventions designed for family members. Family members must be supported to relinquish perceptions that consider family members with mental retardation as childlike and asexual and encouraged to consider sexual expression as part of normal developmental behavior (Dickerson, 1981). Parents, in particular, worry about their children's vulnerabilities even as they participate in the planning for more independent lives within the community (David, Smith, & Friedman, 1976) and interventions such as support groups designed to reduce these anxieties are critical. Additional interventions directed at helping parents to prepare in a concrete manner both within the family and the community for the sexual activities of their children are essential. These interventions might include the provision of formal sex education as well as accessibility to reliable family planning measures.

As a society, our values change slowly. It is important to have an appreciation for this cultural lag when understanding the persistence of narrow and restrictive ideas about mental retardation which are so contradicted by the actual lives lived by many individuals with the disability. Equally important, the so-called progress that seems to characterize the decades since the 1960s cannot be presumed to be self-sustaining. History is not linear and the optimism that was so characteristic of the mid-nineteenth-century field of professionals was replaced by the pessimism of the eugenics movement. Advocacy must be the constant tool used to expand societal concepts about mental retardation as well as to resist regressive forces that seek to limit the full exercise of rights, including sexual expression, by this minority.

REFERENCES

Abel, T., & Kinder, E. (1942). *The subnormal adolescent girl.* New York: Columbia University Press.

Barr, M. W. (1976). The imperative call of our present to our future. In M. Rosen, G. R. Clark, & M. S. Kivitz (Ed.), *The History of Mental Retardation: Collected Papers* (Vol. 2, pp. 99-104). Baltimore: University Park Press.

Brockett, L. P. (1976). Idiots and the efforts for their improvemnent. In M. Rosen, G. R. Clark, & M. S. Kivitz (Ed.), *The History of Mental Retardation: Collected Papers* (Vol. 1, pp. 69-86). Baltimore: University Park Press.

Cegelka, P., & Prehm, H. (1982). *Mental retardation.* London: Charles E. Merrill.

David, H. P., Smith, J. D., & Friedman, E. (1976). Family planning services for persons handicapped by mental retardation. *American Journal Public Health, 66* (11), 1053-1057.

Deutsch, A. (1949). *The mentally ill in America: A history of their care and treatment from colonial times.* New York: Columbia University Press.

Devine, E. (1912). *The family and social work.* New York: Survey Associates.

Dickerson, M. U. (1981). *Social work practice with the mentally retarded.* New York: The Free Press.

Dickin, K. L., & Ryan, B. A. (1983). Sterilization and the mentally retarded. *Canada's Mental Health, 31* (1), 4-8.

Edgerton, R. (1967). *The cloak of competence.* Berkeley: University of California Press.

Edgerton, R. (1979). *Mental retardation.* Cambridge, MA: Harvard University Press.
Farber, B. (1968). *Mental retardation: Its social context and social consequences.* Boston: Houghton Mifflin Company.
Heshusius, Lous. (1981). *Meaning in life as experienced by persons labeled retarded in a group home.* Springfield, IL: Charles C Thomas.
Howe, S. G. (1976). On the causes of idiocy. In M. Rosen, G. R. Clark, & M. S. Kivitz (Eds.), *The history of mental retardation: Collected papers* (Vol. 1, pp. 31-60). Baltimore: University Park Press.
Irvine, A. C. (1988). Balancing the right of the mentally retarded to obtain a therapeutic sterilization against the potential for abuse. *Law & Psychology Review, 12,* 95-122.
Kanner, L. (1949) *A miniature textbook of feeblemindedness.* New York: Child Care Publications.
Macklin, R., & Gaylin, W. (Eds). (1981). *Mental retardation and sterilization: A problem of competency and paternalism.* New York: Plenum Press.
Melton, G. B., & Scott, E. S. (1984). Evaluation of mentally retarded persons for sterilization: Contributions and limits of psychological consultation. *Professional Psychology: Research and Practice, 15* (1), 34-48.
Meyers, R. (1978). *Like normal people.* New York: McGraw Hill.
Monat, R. K. (1982). *Sexuality and the mentally retarded.* San Diego: College-Hill Press.
Nirje, B. (1976). The normalization principle and its human management implications. In M. Rosen, G. R. Clark, & M. S. Kivitz (Eds.), *The history of mental retardation: Collected papers* (Vol. 2, pp. 361-376). Baltimore: University Park Press.
Passer, A., Rauh, J., Chamberlain, A., McGrath, M., & Burket, R. (1984). Issues in fertility control for mentally retarded female adolescents: II. Parental attitudes toward sterilization. *Pediatrics, 73,* 451-454.
Pim, J. (1976). On the necessity of a state provision for the education of the deaf and dumb, the blind and the imbecile. In M. Rosen, G. R. Clark, & M. S. Kivitz (Eds.), *The history of mental retardation: Collected papers* (Vol. 1, pp. 87-101). Baltimore: University Park Press.
Potter, H., & McCollister, C. (1976). A resume of parole work at Letchworth Village. In M. Rosen, G. R. Clark, & M. S. Kivitz (Eds.), *The history of mental retardation: Collected papers* (Vol 2, pp. 127-143). Baltimore: University Park Press.
Rosen, M., Clark, G. R., & Kivitz, M. S. (Eds.). (1976). *The history of mental retardation: Collected papers* (Vol. 2). Baltimore: University Park Press.
Scheerenberger, R. (1983). *A history of mental retardation.* Baltimore: Paul H. Brookes.
Scheerenberger, R. (1987). *A history of mental retardation: A quarter century of promise.* Baltimore: Paul H. Brookes.
Sloan, W., & Stevens, H. (1976). *A century of concern: A history of the American*

Association on Mental Deficiency 1876-1976. Washington, D. C.: American Association on Mental Deficiency.

Stroman, D. (1989). *Mental retardation in social context*. Lanham, MD. University Press of America.

Tyor, P. (1977). "Denied the power to choose the good": Sexuality and mental defect in American medical practice, 1850-1920. *Journal of Social History, 10*, 472-489.

Tyor, P., & Bell, L. (1984). *Caring for the retarded in America*. Westport, CT: Greenwood Press.

Vecoli, R. (1960). Sterilization: A Progressive measure? *Wisconsin Magazine of History, 43*, 190-202.

White, W. D., & Wolfensberger, W. (1969). The evolution of dehumanization in our institutions. *Mental Retardation, 7*, 5-9.

Responding to the Sexual Concerns of Persons with Disabilities

Carol Sandowski

SUMMARY. Sexual messages bombard us daily, yet in professional settings the topic of sexuality is often ignored or is a cause for discomfort. Illness or disability can cause people to feel unattractive and sexually undesirable, but social workers can be instrumental in helping patients and clients by affirming their sexuality. This paper addresses sexual issues facing persons with disabilities and illness and discusses strategies for social workers to assist these clients with their sexual concerns.

In our society certain aspects of life are regarded as private and are often avoided in conversations. Young children learn that it is not polite to ask the age or income of an adult. Discomfort with death is manifest in the use of such terms as, "he passed away," rather than "he died." Likewise, because it is so sensitive many adults avoid serious or personal discussions of sexuality. Social workers counsel individuals and couples on a wide range of issues including such personal matters as finances, grief, and age-associated events such as the "mid-life crisis," but are often reticent to counsel people about sexual matters. In general, sexuality tends to be ignored by most people, including professionals from various disciplines (Kinsey, Pomeroy & Martin, 1948; Kinsey, Pomeroy, Martin & Gebhard, 1953).

In recent years, however, we have witnessed certain exceptions or trends. The frequency with which sexuality is dealt in the media is one example. Another is the recognition and attention given to sexual abuse, in general, and incest in particular. A few years ago it was generally assumed that incest was such a taboo in nearly all cultures that it was virtually non-existent. Professionals and the lay public now know that incest is a problem of great magnitude. It is being addressed by both therapists and survivors. Denying the existence of sexuality following a disability is reminiscent of denying incest in past years. As more people with disabilities express their concerns over sexual issues and more professionals inquire if they have sexual problems and get affirmative responses, there is realization that these concerns have always existed. This discussion will address ways in which professionals can assist persons with disabilities with their sexual concerns.

Among the most sexually outspoken are young people with disabilities. This is particularly true for persons with spinal cord injuries who, prior to their injuries, have led physically active lives vocationally, recreationally, and sexually. They have questions about their future lives and are vocal in expressing concerns and seeking answers. Likewise, individuals with multiple sclerosis and diabetes also tend to express their feelings of frustration, particularly since their sexual functioning tends to be affected while their libido remains intact. Persons with disabilities who are willing to express their feelings are likely to experience great relief when social workers or other professionals affirm them as sexual beings with normal needs and desires.

Other people with disabilities seem to struggle along in relative silence. Studies of stroke survivors indicate that frequency of sexual relations decreases following stroke though sexual desire and capacity for sexual functioning remains basically unchanged (Grady, DeFrank & Wolfe, 1981; Renshaw, 1978; Sjogren & Fugl-Meyer, 1981). Since strokes occur predominantly among the elderly, it may be that those who suffer strokes are more resigned and accepting of such changes as something that comes with age. Perhaps, discomfort inhibits them from asking or talking about sexual issues. It may also be that their health and human services providers do not provide them an opportunity to discuss sexual concerns.

Persons with Parkinson's Disease are similar in age to stroke survivors, and as a group, they, too, tend to be reticent about discussing sexual issues. Even though one out of every one hundred persons over the age of sixty is affected by the disease, very little research exists on the effects of Parkinson's Disease on sexuality. More research is needed to increase our knowledge. At one time, for example, it was thought that L-dopa had the quality of an aphrodisiac because persons with Parkinson's, given this medication, showed renewed interest and vigor in sexual activity. However, it is more likely to be as Esibill (1983) contends that sexual interest and activity increase because L-dopa produces greater comfort and function.

In researching the effects of Parkinson's Disease on sexuality the author (Sandowski, 1989) was left with many unanswered questions. Is the dearth of research on Parkinson's because this older, less verbal population seems to no longer care about sexual relations? Or is it because researchers and other health professionals assume they no longer care? Is the lack of sexual interest for persons with Parkinson's related to depression or to brain chemistry? How important are social factors in affecting intimacy in long term relationships? For example, when the person with Parkinson's Disease appears serious and unsmiling, does the partner respond as though the patient was unloving and uncaring rather than the innocent carrier of the facial mask associated with Parkinson's Disease? These questions illustrate the need for more research in the area of sexuality and Parkinson's Disease. Similar research related to stroke and other medical and disabling conditions is also needed.

It is clear that persons with disabilities are sexual beings with needs and desires for intimacy. One can not assume that people who avoid the topic of sexuality lack sexual feelings, desires, or concerns (Masters & Johnson, 1966). Instead, environments in which clients can feel comfortable talking about sexuality can be created. For example, a tactful statement suggesting that one is available to discuss any sexual concerns may very well be appreciated by a person with a disability. Social workers can minimize individuals' struggles with issues of sexuality by improving practice settings and providing sexual counseling. In addition, further sexual research is needed to provide understanding of the effects of disability on sexual functioning.

DEALING WITH SEXUALITY IN MEDICAL SETTINGS

Often sexuality seems to be ignored in medical settings, though social workers have opportunities to rectify this situation. There seem to be several legitimate reasons why the subject of sexuality is ignored in hospital and rehabilitation settings. People with medical conditions typically have numerous questions that need answering at the time of the diagnosis or injury and throughout the recovery process. Sexuality may be less urgent than immediate medical crises. In addition, some people are too intimidated to inquire about sexual matters. Others may feel they should be able to resolve personal matters on their own. If they do raise questions related to their sexuality, they may find that helping professionals lack answers or may be too embarrassed to respond appropriately. Sometimes patients may be too depressed to even care about issues of intimacy. Some couples may feel hopeless and believe there are no solutions to their sexual problems, especially if social workers and health care providers do not tell them otherwise.

Health care providers may ignore sexuality because they are reluctant to intrude upon patients' personal lives or because their discomfort prohibits them from making inquiries. However other circumstances must be considered. In the author's social work experience working in a rehabilitation facility, the major deterrents to offering sexual counseling are lack of time and privacy. Privacy is limited by all the distractions and intrusions of semi-private rooms. Patients, seen at the time of admission, are often accompanied not only by spouses, but by adult-aged children, other relatives, or close friends. Informing newly admitted patients and their spouses that sexual counseling is available can be difficult. Timing may also present difficulties. Patients and family members are typically anxious at the time of admission and have many questions. Closer to discharge, anxiety again mounts as patients and families prepare to leave a safe, helpful, and supportive environment. There are questions about the need for further therapy, equipment, and managing in one's familiar home with a still unfamiliar body.

From the time of admission until discharge the patient's energy is typically directed towards physical, occupational and other therapies, medical management and possibly nursing care. The spouse's or partner's energy, meanwhile, is channeled towards hospital visits, meeting normal obligations, and performing duties usually assumed by the hospitalized partner. The social worker, in the meantime, juggles various team meetings with a full caseload of patients and rushes to meet the inevitable crisis situations that occur almost daily with the result being that issues of sexuality may not be a high priority.

In comprehensive rehabilitation facilities, most aspects of a person's life are evaluated and treated during the rehabilitation process. Even issues unrelated or indirectly related to one's health may be scrutinized. For example, a driver's evaluation can be done to determine if the patient will be safe driving again, or if adaptive automobile equipment is needed for driving. Yet when it comes to sexual functioning, too many patients are on their own to find out what they can or cannot do.

Certainly sexuality is such a private matter that some people would prefer to be left alone to discover their capabilities in the privacy of their own homes, and their wishes should be respected. Others, however, are relieved when someone raises the topic. A social worker can offer help in the form of reassurance, encouragement, and specific information. Social workers have the unique opportunity to be available in a wide range of settings: acute care hospitals, rehabilitation facilities, various clinics, and home health agencies. In addition to medical settings, there are mental health and private practice settings. Oftentimes, patients' concerns surface only after they return home from inpatient care, thus social workers who follow patients after discharge or work with home health agencies may be in an ideal position to provide sexual counseling.

While it is generally agreed that responding to patients' sexual concerns is an important part of physical rehabilitation, the reality is that not all facilities provide structured programs. For many patients, the extent of dealing with sexual problems is limited to doctors and nurses answering questions, or social workers, psychologists, or even chaplains providing limited sexual counseling within counseling sessions that deal with a wide range of adjustment issues. For social workers to be effective in providing adequate sexual counseling, they need to acquire an understanding of how disability impacts on sexuality and they must make counseling a priority. Often this requires obtaining institutional support and frequently necessitates specialized professional training.

Miller, Szasz, and Anderson (1981) describe in detail the role of a sexual health care clinician and a hospital administrator's decision to create a sexual health care service (SHCS) as a distinct, specialized hospital service. This program requires that the clinician's work begin shortly after admission to the acute unit and follow patients through their stay in the rehabilitation center. Occasionally it involves follow-up appointments related to specific concerns such as fertility. The sexual health care clinician's responsibilities involve patient services, staff inservices and education, liaison with hospital and community agencies, and administration and research. The clinician is a member of the team and, as such, attends team meetings, but the clinician is also directly responsible to the physician clinical director of SHCS. Though most settings do not have the luxury of a comprehensive program as just described, with social work initiative, sexual counseling programs can be developed methodically, with new elements of the program added gradually.

Staff development with an emphasis on in-services to help staff to feel comfortable with personal and patient sexuality is an important first step. Informing patients that sexual counseling is available could be done briefly in the introductory packets of information often given to patients and their families at the time of admission. The message, "Sex is spoken here," is conveyed. Availability of trained staff to offer counseling when needed and a referral process for such services is, of course, essential. In this way, sexual counseling is available "upon request." As staff knowledge and skill increases, more services can be added.

The reality is that social workers will, at times, be called on to address issues of sexuality with their patients and clients. Prepared social workers will feel comfortable, if not with sexual counseling, then with making appropriate referrals. Ideally, social workers will develop expertise and facilitate program development to address the spectrum of patient sexuality needs.

SEXUAL COUNSELING

Social workers interested in developing sexual counseling skills can obtain the necessary training from sexual training programs, professional consultation, and personal study. As they acquire knowledge and skills, their abilities to help with clients' sexual concerns expand.

The PLISSIT model of sexual counseling, developed by Annon (1976) is used extensively by professionals who engage in sexual counseling and provides a useful intervention framework that lends itself well to medical settings. Visually depicted, it has a triangular shape. At the broad base is the "P" of "PLISSIT," which represents "permission-giving." Most health care professionals acknowledge that sexuality is a natural, normal part of life and accept that individuals with disabilities have sexual feelings and sexual concerns, and it is reassuring for patients and clients to hear this. By so doing, the message is conveyed that it is permissible to talk about sex.

The next level up, "limited information" (LI) requires more knowledge and skill. In this narrower portion of the symbolic triangle most, but not all health care professionals can offer some general, non-technical information. It may simply mean telling the patient that he or she is not alone–that others have expressed similar feelings. Or it might involve advice to a couple to find different, more comfortable positions during sexual intimacy. Nurses and others may be asked questions by patients while tending to patients' personal needs, or by visiting spouses. For example, one patient's spouse assumed that her husband's catheter signalled the end of their sex lives. She was reassured to learn that this assumption was incorrect and was further relieved to learn the catheter was temporary. This limited information did much to alleviate the wife's anxiety.

Proceeding up towards the point of the triangle, is "specific suggestions" (SS). Suggestions are made by those who are knowledgeable and have sufficient counseling skills to provide information with sensitivity. The social worker or other professional considers the patient's or client's preferences and previous lifestyle when offering counsel. A nurse offering specific suggestions may advise a couple on how to manage a catheter during intercourse, or how to minimize the likelihood of a bowel or bladder accident. A social worker may help a couple by offering specific suggestions on how to improve sexual communication. For those couples who have never discussed their sexual likes and dislikes, the social worker's encouragement to do so will help them adapt to changes brought about by the illness or disability.

At the apex of the triangle is "intensive therapy" (IT). As the name suggests, this level involves sexual therapy by a trained sex therapist. This would involve taking a sexual history and seeing the patient or client with his or her partner. It may involve marital therapy or dealing with other issues such as past sexual traumas like incest or rape.

The PLISSIT model clearly shows that all providers can deal with sexual issues but to different degrees. All professionals can provide "Permission" (P), even those who lack specialized sexuality training. Increasing comfort, knowledge, and skill is necessary as one approaches the need for "Intensive Therapy" (IT). When professionals reach their limits they can refer patients to colleagues who are better qualified to respond to specific patient concerns.

CONSIDERATIONS IN COUNSELING PERSONS WITH ILLNESS AND DISABILITY

Clients with disabilities or health problems often have concerns and needs that require special attention. Occasionally clients have called the author requesting sexual counseling after having been turned down by other sex therapists who said that they did not work with persons with disabilities. Certainly it is important for each social worker to identify the client population he or she works with best, and recognize personal and professional strengths and limitations. Those who work with persons with chronic illnesses or disabilities must be willing to learn about special needs and develop the skills necessary to be of help to clients.

As with any sexual counseling, taking a sexual history to determine client needs and to plan interventions, is a crucial first step when counseling persons with disabilities. For example, people with medical conditions from birth, such as cerebral palsy, are likely to have somewhat different life experiences because opportunities may be limited. Concerns of the person with a life-long disability may center on the need to be recognized as a sexual person or on the question of how to meet potential partners. An adequate sexual history helps the social worker identify and respond to specific client concerns.

Competently prepared social workers who take sexual histories are mindful of psychological and physical factors and how they interact. When indicated, they refer clients for medical consultation. For example, in assessing the causes of erectile dysfunction, it is generally thought that sudden onset of impotence is more likely to be the result of psychological factors whereas gradual onset tends to be caused by physical problems. A thorough examination by a urologist with specialized knowledge of erectile dysfunction can determine if there is a physical cause of the problem. Similarly, a gynecologist, advised of a female patient's symptoms, can determine if there is a physical basis for symptoms such as dryness (lack of lubrication) or painful intercourse.

Other considerations when counseling persons affected by illness or disability are discussed below.

Self-Image

A major aspect of counseling involves addressing client self-esteem. When illness or disability strikes, self-esteem can be seriously assaulted. For example, when a patient told the author he "feels like a leper" since being diagnosed with cancer he underscored just how important self-esteem issues are. In a medical setting, the social worker can facilitate the cooperation of other professionals who can help patients regain their sense of self-worth. When nurses assist with routine grooming activities, a cheerful, positive approach can convey messages of "You are important." Helping or encouraging patients to get a haircut, apply make-up, or splash on a bit of cologne helps patients look and feel better. In a subtle way, there is an unspoken message that, "You are important and deserve this for yourself." The patient's self-worth and sexual well-being are likely to be enhanced. Within the rehabilitation setting, occupational therapists also promote grooming and independence in all daily living skills (ADL's). Fostering independence not only enhances one's self-esteem but also helps relationships that are often strained by the patient's many needs.

It is important to send credible messages. For example, when doctors and nurses tell ostomy patients that their healing stoma looks "beautiful," patients are likely to react with disbelief. Perhaps it would be more accurate to acknowledge, "You may not think so, but I think the stoma looks great!" or simply, "The stoma is healing nicely, and looks just the way it should." That the appearance is at least "normal" may be of some comfort. Each day, many people, professionals as well as family and friends convey messages to patients verbally and non-verbally. How these messages are sent and perceived will have an effect on the patient's altered self-image, and subsequently his or her self-esteem. When an individual feels good about him or herself, it will be reflected in the quality of intimate relationships.

Adjustment

Grief stems from any major loss including loss of health, functioning, or independence and both patients and their partners go through a grieving process. Illness or a disabling condition may result in an altered lifestyle and role changes for both partners. The unaffected partner may be forced to take on many of the duties of the one who is no longer able to perform customary tasks. The partner may feel ignored or forgotten at the very time when he or she is feeling overburdened physically, emotionally, and financially. The social worker can help by providing supportive counseling, education and information, and referrals to local support groups or other community resources. Social work involvement may enable either or both partners to cope better by helping them to identify their primary concerns, establish priorities, delegate tasks, or delay any stressful major decisions that can be postponed.

Physical Concerns and Intimate Relationships

Social workers can be instrumental in helping couples communicate openly and honestly. Even couples with rich and varied sex lives may need help to discuss sexuality related feelings and preferences. For some couples the onset of a medical condition means it is necessary to discuss and plan for sexual activity rather than expect the spontaneous sex they may have previously had.

Some patients require considerable assistance with personal needs. This can be a physical burden for spouses, but more than that, it is often difficult for partners to provide personal care such as bowel and bladder management and also act as spouses and lovers. Some partners, especially when the disability is severe, find care-giving demands overwhelming. Some are distressed by specific personal care activities. Often the solution is to obtain outside help so that the roles of caretaker and lover are kept separate. Information that hired help for caretaking activities is available and can be beneficial to the relationship may make this option acceptable.

Sexual relationships may be affected by medications, such as anti-hypertensives and anti-depressants. Some medications diminish libido while others cause erectile dysfunction in males and lack of lubrication in females. Physicians can review the patient medications to assess their sexual impact and, if needed, prescribe different medications or modify dosages. Social workers and other health professionals can encourage patients to discuss their medications with their physicians, and can help patients to find ways to coordinate sexual activity with time of medication. For example, some are able to have sex in the morning before taking their first dose of medicine. Social workers can also help people understand the dangers of altering dosages or discontinuing medications without consulting their physicians.

For some patients, it is helpful to offer advice or suggestions related to positions to use during sexual activity. For example, couples who have always had sexual relations in the "missionary" position may need to experiment in order to find more comfortable positions. In some cases it may be helpful to get input from a physical or occupational therapist for clients who have complications such as muscle spasms or contractures.

Persons who experience pain from conditions such as arthritis or chronic back pain will also benefit from finding comfortable positions for lovemaking. Then their partners can accommodate accordingly while allowing those who experience pain to have freedom of movement and the ability to move away if necessary. For some it may be advantageous to schedule sexual activity for those times when pain medication is working at a peak, or after having been up and walking about for awhile in the morning.

Fear can also interfere with a satisfying sexual relationship. The fear of being unable to "perform," the fear of experiencing or causing pain or the fear that one's partner or oneself will have a recurrent heart attack or stroke may be serious deterrents to feelings of sexual desire. Social work intervention to reduce fear involves listening to the patient or client and providing reassurance and education. For example, it is usually standard practice to advise cardiac patients that sex is safe as long as the patient is able to walk up a flight or two of stairs without problems. Stroke survivors can be assured that, with blood pressure under control, they are safe to have sex. Some people benefit from being informed that they will not contract conditions like cancer from partners who have cancer (Schover, 1988). Accurate information can ameliorate many fears clients present.

Whatever the sexual adjustment issue, the social worker can positively influence the self image and intimate lives of patients, their partners, and families. For many patients, hospitalization and the onset of a life-changing medical or disabling condition result in their very first contact with a social worker. As social workers address psychosocial needs, services may vary widely and include counseling, facilitating referrals, and providing concrete services such as discharge planning. Sexuality needs of clients and partners may be a particularly important point of intervention for social workers as they identify needs, provide counseling, consult with physicians, and when necessary, facilitate referrals.

Indicators of Outcome

The desire for specific and concrete answers to questions about sexual abilities is not uncommon. Questions, however, may be "loaded" with multiple meanings. For example, the question, "Will I be able to have children?" may also mean, "Will I be able to have sex?" It may also mean, "Will anyone find me attractive or sexually desirable?" A social worker with sexual counseling skills can search for the multiple meanings and help patients deal with these issues.

Information is not always easy to provide, however. For example, a thorough neurological examination of a person with a spinal cord injury can predict, fairly accurately, the individual's sexual potential, nevertheless such predictions are tentative and only time will prove or disprove diagnostic accuracy in individual cases. With the brain as the core of one's sexuality, even serious conditions need not be sexually devastating. For example, spinal cord injuries cause profound changes in sexual functioning, yet individuals with spinal cord injuries and their partners can have satisfying sexual lives. Pleasurable sensations are altered, but are still possible. In some instances, individuals find that their bodies seem to compensate for lack of genital sensation; often areas above the lesion are intensely and sensuously responsive to touch. Even with absent genital sensation, some persons with spinal cord injuries are able to experience orgasms. Others may be anorgasmic but still enjoy pleasuring their partners and being touched, pleasured and caressed by their partners in non-genital areas they can feel and even in genital areas they cannot feel.

Overall, the best indicators of client sexual adjustment are the willingness of providers to discuss sexuality and sexual adjustment with clients and their partners, combined with client desires for intimacy and willingness to address sexual concerns. Ideally, social workers will be able to answer questions and provide information to maximize sexual outcomes and enhance intimate relationships.

CONCLUDING REMARKS

Knowledge about human sexual functioning and identification of the psychological and physical factors that can interfere with sexual functioning for males and females has increased. There are also more treatment options available, particularly for physical problems. As people live longer and are more likely to be affected by disabilities or chronic medical conditions, it is important that we understand what impact these can have on all areas of a person's life. Social workers can obtain valuable training and insights into the needs and coping mechanisms of individuals and couples who are dealing with illness or disability. A willingness to provide sexual counseling is a valuable service that enables couples to experience an improved quality of life.

Given the fact that many professionals have had inadequate sex education themselves, it is understandable that some social workers and other professionals have avoided sexual counseling. Ideally, more schools of social work will offer courses in human sexuality in order to better prepare social workers for dealing with the numerous sexual problems of the 1990s. Conferences, seminars, and other continuing education programs are also valuable.

Social workers who feel comfortable providing sexual counseling may feel inadequate in dealing with clients who have particular medical conditions. If so, it is important to assess the knowledge and skills they need in order to be effective. Such preparation will help the therapist feel more confident in providing services their clients need. To enhance their skills, social workers can obtain additional information from various sources including physician consultation, literature searches, and professional supervision. In addition, organizations such as the National Spinal Cord Injury Association, the National Stroke Association, or the American Cancer Society are excellent resources and can provide information and referrals.

Research and knowledge in the scientific study of sexuality is very new. While technology is providing us with cures and treatments, it is still important that individuals and couples receive adequate counseling that enables them to know and explore the full range of options available to them. Despite technical advances, many couples are relieved to learn that it is possible to enhance their intimate relationships without resorting to surgery or costly medical treatment.

For professionals working in the field of sexuality and disability, it is an exciting time of continued growth and learning, not just in the classroom but in our work with clients. In her concluding remarks to a group of professionals at Marianjoy Rehabilitation Center, Dr. Domeena Renshaw, founder and director of the Sexual Dysfunction Clinic at Loyola Hospital since 1972, said, "We learn from our patients and our clients. They are our textbooks."

Social workers have a responsibility to deal holistically with their clients who have disabilities. This includes acknowledging clients' sexual concerns and affirming them as sexual beings. The social worker's presence, support and counseling while clients explore issues of intimacy can be as healing as advice that is offered. Sexual feelings, needs, and desires may exist into the final years of a person's life, even when illness or disability strikes. Social workers, who work to enhance their clients' quality of life in so many ways, can aid clients in ways that have been ignored for too long.

REFERENCES

Annon, J. S. (1976). *Behavioral treatment of sexual problems: Brief therapy.* New York: Harper & Row, Pub., Inc.

Esibill, N. (1983). Impact of Parkinson's disease on sexuality. *Sexuality and Disability, 6,* 120-125.

Grady, P. B, DeFrank, R. S., & Wolfe, T. L. (1981). Sexual functioning in stroke survivors. *Archives of Physical Medicine and Rehabilitation, 62,* 286-88.

Kinsey, A. C., Pomeroy, W. B., & Martin, C. E. (1948). *Sexual behavior in the human male.* Philadelphia: W. B. Saunders.

Kinsey, A. C., Pomeroy, W. B., Martin, C. E., & Gebhard, P. H. (1953). *Sexual behavior in the human female,* Philadelphia: W. B. Saunders.

Masters, W. H., & Johnson, V. E. (1966). *Human sexual response.* Boston: Little, Brown & Co.

Miller S., Szasz G., & Anderson L. (1981). Sexual health care clinician in an acute spinal cord injury unit. *Archives of Physical Medicine and Rehabilitation, 62,* 315-320.

Renshaw, D. C. (1978). Stroke and sex. In A. Comfort (Ed.), *Sexual consequences of disability.* Philadelphia: George F. Stickley Company.

Sandowski, C. (1989). *Sexual concerns when illness or disability strikes.* Springfield, IL: Charles C Thomas, Publishing.

Schover, L. R. (1988). *Sexuality and cancer.* American Cancer Society, Inc., p. 28.

Sjogren K., & Fugl-Meyer, A. R. (1981). Sexual problems in hemiplegia. *International Rehabilitation Medicine, 3,* 26-31.

Training in Sexuality and Disability: Preparing Social Workers to Provide Services to Individuals with Disabilities

Pamela S. Boyle

SUMMARY. Millions of people in our society have disabilities. Social workers are often looked upon to provide these individuals and their significant others with guidance and counseling related to matters of sexuality, intimacy and personal relationships. To be adequately prepared to do this, it is important that social workers be in touch with their personal values and beliefs, that they have factual information about sexuality and disability, and that they possess the skills to convey positive attitudes and knowledge to their clients. This paper, therefore, presents a staff development program that trains professionals to help their clients with disabilities develop positive sexual self-images and to aid them in establishing full social and sexual lives.

Ideally, social workers would be knowledgeable, skilled and sensitive to issues related to sexuality and disability when they leave college and university programs. They would take this knowledge, these skills and this sensitivity into practice settings where they would find individuals in great need of the sexual guidance they have to offer. More specifically, they would routinely provide sex education, sex counseling and advocacy services to persons with disabilities (Goldsmith, 1979). Unfortunately, social workers often lack training and expertise, yet people expect counselors and therapists to assist them with an understanding of issues of intimacy and sexuality and offer help and guidance (Brashear, 1978).

The purpose of this article is to outline three basic components of staff training related to sexuality and disability for hospital, habilitation or rehabilitation facilities. Suggestions are intended to assist social workers who are responsible for or who desire to develop this kind of staff training program and to supplement the knowledge of those who may already have this kind of training.

Unfortunately, social workers and other professionals providing services to people with disabilities are often unprepared to deal with issues of sexuality and intimacy, whether these disabilities are physical, cognitive or sensory in nature. In formal education programs for social workers, rehabilitation counselors and others in training to provide direct counseling and education services to people with disabilities, the issue of sexuality is given scant attention by instructors who are themselves underprepared to provide instruction to tomorrow's professionals (Chubon, 1981). The author's experiences in graduate school reflect this description. Discussions related to self-concept, self-esteem, adjustment to an altered body image and other such topics stopped short of dealing directly and openly with the sexual concerns which individuals with disabilities often have. Many rehabilitation counselors leave an otherwise exceptional program of training without the knowledge and skills to answer questions and address the needs of individuals related to issues of human sexuality. This has been the experience of many individuals in professional schools (Brashear, 1978). It still remains the experience of many students in 1992.

Given the lack of training and education at the college and university level and the demand for sexuality services by individuals with disabilities, Sexual Attitude Reassessment Programs (SARs) were sponsored by several of the major rehabilitation centers around the country (Chipouras, 1979). Participants included people with and without disabilities. SAR training experiences generally began on a Friday night and concluded on Sunday afternoon. The experience included small and large group work, a wide array of films, short lectures and panel discussions. The SAR experience was one few participants forgot. It was very often their first opportunity to openly discuss thoughts, experiences, feelings and questions about sexuality and individuals with disabilities. Sexual Attitude Reassessment Programs are no longer readily available in all areas of the country despite the fact that they provided an excellent opportunity for learning. Budget constraints in programs and facilities and the changing political and religious climate probably contributed to the discontinuance of some SARs. It is, therefore, incumbent on habilitation and rehabilitation programs to plan in-house training opportunities for staff.

Sexuality can be defined as the integration of physical, emotional, intellectual and psychological aspects of an individual's personality which express maleness or femaleness (Chipouras, Cornelius, Daniels & Makas, 1979). Sexuality in its broadest sense is expressed in most of the circumstances in which an individual finds herself or himself on a daily basis: socializing, working, discussions of religion or politics, and raising children. Sexuality is a part of our identity and is as much a part of who we are as what we do. Typical discussions about sexuality in our society, however, are performance oriented and involve discussions about sexual acts, sexual function/dysfunction, beauty, size and satisfaction. Frequently, a performance oriented view of sexuality focuses on deficits. The notion that individuals with disabilities are sexual and have sexuality needs is frequently denied. With these dominant views of sexuality in our culture, the sexuality needs of people with disabilities tend to be neglected or controlled.

Social workers and other human service providers, simply by virtue of their caring nature, are not necessarily exempt from these attitudes. Staff training programs are essential if we are to provide professionals with the opportunity to examine their attitudes, values and beliefs related to both issues of sexuality, and sexuality and disability. They must also gain factual knowledge about sexuality and sexuality and disability and improve and acquire skills in the provision of direct services to individuals with disabilities and their significant others.

Three components of a staff training program on sexuality and disability will be described. The first of these components relates to sexual attitudes, values and beliefs, how they develop and what effect they have on providers of sexuality information and guidance. Secondly, staff training includes a body of factual information which relates to sexuality in general, and more specifically to sexual issues of concern to specific populations of individuals served by the practitioners in the training group. Finally, the program of training provides skill development which increases the social worker's ability to routinely offer basic sexuality education and guidance to their clients.

TRAINING DIRECTED AT PARTICIPANT ATTITUDES, VALUES AND BELIEFS

Most people have had few opportunities to seriously discuss issues of sexuality in their personal lives or within academic environments. It is easy to joke about sexual matters, but serious discussion of the issues is often accompanied by feelings of discomfort (Brashear, 1978). The first portion of a staff training opportunity should be devoted to increasing the participants' abilities to deal with issues of sexuality commonly raised by their clients by reducing their own levels of anxiety related to sexual matters. This can be accomplished through the use of both experiential exercises and discussions of values and feelings that emerge. There are several good sources for this type of material (Hartman, Quinn, and Young, 1981; Valois and Kammerman, 1984; Morrison and Underhill Price, 1974; Simon, Howe and Kirschenbaum, 1972). Planned Parenthood affiliates may also be able to provide information and suggestions.

Exercises used in training should be chosen carefully and with clear purpose. Exercises should be scheduled in ways that respect individual readiness and group processes. Exercises requiring the least self-disclosure, generating little anxiety may be presented early in the group process. As participants feel more comfortable with both the topic and other group members, more emotionally and interpersonally challenging exercises can be introduced. Some level of self-disclosure is necessary; increasing self-awareness and exploring feelings and attitudes are helpful if participants are to increase their capacity to deal with sexuality in daily contact with clients (Chubon, 1981). While personal information will most likely be shared with others in the training group, this part of the training does not demand that participants self-disclose to the point of discomfort.

This portion of training is not intended to force participants to change their attitudes, values or beliefs related to either sexuality or more specifically, sexuality and disability. The purpose is to assist and guide participants in the process of determining how their attitudes and values may affect their interactions with their clients, while increasing their level of comfort with sexuality. This portion of the training is generally very interactive and enjoyable. Some participants may feel uncomfortable speaking about sexuality in such an open forum; however, most participants appreciate the opportunity to share their thoughts and feelings. Exposing sexual myths and misinformation and identifying family, societal and cultural influences are favorite topics of most participants. This part of the training program allows participants to reflect and sometimes laugh at the knowledge and attitudes they learned as children and may still possess as adults and professionals. It is exceptionally important for the facilitator to model openness by appropriately using self-disclosure to promote discussion.

One exercise that can be used to promote group cohesiveness and begin the process of self-disclosure among members is entitled "Early Influences–Current Attitudes about Sexuality."

Early Influences–Current Attitudes
About Sexuality

In the large group, the trainer asks the participants to consider the following three questions:

1. Remember your earliest years as a child and as a teenager. Who provided you with your first information about sex?
2. What were your reactions to this information? How did you feel?
3. Who or what do you think most influenced your current sexual attitudes?

The trainer should ask the participants to think about these questions and their answers for approximately ten minutes. The trainer may ask participants to jot down their thoughts on paper if it is available.

After participants have had an opportunity to consider their answers, the trainer divides the large group into dyads or triads. The participants are instructed to share their responses within their small group for approximately ten minutes. The trainer should be clear, however, that participants should share only that information or those feelings with which they feel comfortable. There should be no demand for more self-disclosure than each participant feels is appropriate. This strategy is an important opportunity for the trainer to model respect for personal pace in the process of discussing issues of sexuality and personal concerns.

After small group interaction, the trainer brings the large group together again. Using newsprint or an overhead projector, the trainer should write responses generated by participants. The "Early Influences–Current Attitudes about Sexuality" exercise generates lively discussion about a wide variety of experiences. Differences between men and women emerge, for example, and religious, cultural and geographical differences often highlight discussions. Participants often emerge from the experience with a better understanding of how one's own past and the past of others influence the present and an increased understanding of how present day influences affect attitudes, values and beliefs about sexuality.

The second portion of the training pertaining to attitudes, values and beliefs includes additional experiential exercises which engage participants in discussions of their beliefs and attitudes related specifically to sexuality and individuals with disabilities. While participants may have positive, non-judgmental attitudes about sexuality for individuals without disabilities, they may be less clear about their feelings related to sexuality for individuals with disabilities (Brashear, 1978). Social workers may presume that sexuality is unimportant to individuals with disabilities. They may never have been asked questions related to the issue. They may also believe that sexuality is too painful for clients to discuss in counseling or that it is or should be the last thing on clients' minds. The social worker may have difficulty understanding how anyone would ever find individuals with physical disabilities desirable as social or sexual partners. Some may believe that individuals with disabilities have "more important things" to be thinking about and that they should simply be "happy to be alive." These attitudes can become evident to clients who may then adopt similar beliefs or become too intimidated to ask about sexuality. All of these issues are discussed early in the training program so that participants can thoroughly examine and overcome stereotypical thoughts or biases they may have toward people with disabilities.

A true and false questionnaire that assesses participant knowledge and attitudes is a useful technique to uncover biases or misunderstandings participants may have toward people with disabilities and their sexuality. The following questionnaire is one example. It is intended only as a suggestion. Trainers should add, delete and modify statements to reflect myths typical of specific disabilities and the participants' level of knowledge and awareness.

Sexuality
and Disabilities Questionnaire

The trainer distributes the following questionnaire to participants with the instructions that each person should respond to each statement with either "true" or "false." The participants should be told that the questionnaires will not be collected and they will not be required to share their answers unless they wish.

1. People with disabilities do not think about sex.
2. Individuals with disabilities are not attractive to people without disabilities.
3. Women marry men with disabilities because they enjoy the role of mother or nurse.
4. People with disabilities are never able to make good parents.
5. A satisfying, intimate relationship does not always include traditional sexual intercourse.
6. A satisfying sexual relationship is as much emotional and psychological as physical.
7. People with disabilities have no sex drive.
8. Marriage is not desired by people with disabilities.
9. It is difficult for people with disabilities to talk about issues of sexuality.
10. People with disabilities are infertile.

After approximately 5-7 minutes, the trainer should lead a discussion addressing each item on the questionnaire to dispel myths and provide accurate information to participants.

Training programs designed for social workers working with individuals with specific disabilities should be adapted to address the specific concerns and issues most relevant and appropriate. For example, participants working with individuals with mental retardation or developmental disabilities (MR/DD) may include discussions clarifying the sexual rights of individuals with developmental disabilities and considering their roles in protecting these basic human rights while protecting a potentially vulnerable population from exploitation. Some participants may worry that raising issues of sexuality with people with mental retardation would create problems that could simply be avoided by ignoring sexuality. Some may see individuals with MR/DD as perpetual children who are likely to be hurt or exploited. Others may feel that the parents of these individuals do not want professionals to enter into sexuality education or training with their sons or daughters.

The training program helps participants to identify client needs, personal values and misconceptions, thus helping them deal with these issues with increased comfort and knowledge. Participant exploration of personal values, attitudes, beliefs, misconceptions and misinformation make for interesting discussions during the first part of training. Values exploration also helps people better understand client needs and increases the likelihood that a commitment to meet those needs will be made. It is necessary for participants to become more self-aware and gain an increased understanding of their own sexuality if they are to benefit fully from the remaining components of training and ultimately translate their learning into improved practice.

INFORMATION AND KNOWLEDGE BUILDING

The second part of a sexuality and disability training workshop should provide factual information related to both general sexuality and to sexuality and disability. Providing factual information does several things. First, having factual information may help social workers feel more comfortable initiating sexuality discussions with clients. Second, it may increase practitioner comfort in handling basic sexuality questions which may be raised in therapeutic relationships. Third, practitioners who participate in the training will be able to offer accurate factual information, not speculation based on an assumption or guessing. Individuals seeking assistance with sexuality issues may have inadequate or inaccurate information. As social workers provide accurate information they demystify sex, correct myths and fallacies, and assist clients to manage their sexual lives more comfortably, safely and with greater personal satisfaction.

The first component of the information and knowledge section of training should deal with issues such as: basic male and female sexual anatomy and physiology, the sexual response cycle, menstruation, contraception and conception, sexual lifestyles and sexual orientation, masturbation and other expressions of sexuality. Given that time for training is often at a premium, the facilitator chooses issues that will be most relevant and of most interest to the group of trainees. Information provided should be basic and practical and should be designed to enrich discussions of sexuality within the therapeutic relationship. The facilitator should be certain to use a variety of teaching resources which include audiovisual materials, models of human genital anatomy, diagrams, pictures, and appropriate handouts. Optimum participant benefit comes from lively and active involvement of all members. The most current literature on human sexuality must be an integral part of the preparation for this part of the training program (Francouer, 1991).

There are several entertaining and interesting ways to impart factual information. "Sexual Jeopardy" can be developed using a large cork board and construction paper. As with the television version, this game includes categories and a series of related "answers," each of which is worth points. The answers worth 100 points should be easier than the questions worth 500 points. Categories may include male anatomy, female anatomy, the sexual response cycle, birth control methods, pregnancy, sexual lifestyles, and sexual development. Participants can be divided into two (or more) teams. Each member of the team takes a turn and chooses a question in one of the categories. If the participant gives the correct answer, his or her team gains points. If the question is incorrectly answered, points are lost. "Daily Double" and a difficult "Final Jeopardy" question (to be answered by the entire team) can be included. At the end of the competition, the team with the most accumulated points "wins." Other methods of imparting sexuality information include crossword puzzles made up of sexuality terms and definitions, basic diagrams of male and female anatomy which can be completed individually or in teams and descriptions with blanks to be filled in with the missing terms.

The second component of the information and knowledge portion of training is disability-specific and is designed to provide basic, factual information about sexual issues which relate to the specific group of clients or patients of concern to the training participants. In a rehabilitation setting, for example, issues of concern to be discussed may include physical disability, chronic illness, and cognitive and behavioral deficits following traumatic brain injury. Participants may want to know answers to questions such as: Just what can a man with a spinal cord injury expect in regard to erection and ejaculation? What are his treatment options regarding difficulty in having erections? What are the effects of closed head injuries both cognitively and behaviorally relative to sex? Is it a good idea for a person who has had a stroke to resume sexual activity? Does this increase the chances of having another stroke? Can a woman with quadriplegia have a baby? If she doesn't want to have a baby, what kind of birth control would she be able to use safely and effectively? What does the individual who uses an indwelling catheter do with it during sexual activity? What are the effects of multiple sclerosis on sexual functioning? Needless to say, the list of potential questions and issues is lengthy. The facilitator will need to be aware of the particular issues which will most likely confront the participants and be prepared to discuss them. There are several excellent resources for this information (Neistadt and Freda, 1987; Schover and Jensen, 1988; Rabin, 1980; Sandowski, 1989; Comfort, 1978; Kempton, 1987; Haavik and Menninger, 1981; Monat, 1982). Participants may have very little factual information about sexuality and specific disabilities. It may be necessary for the trainer to provide "mini-lectures" with relevant handouts or use audio-visuals to provide information. For example, participants in the workshop who serve individuals with developmental disabilities may be concerned with such issues as: informed consent; attitudes of parents of individuals with mental retardation or other developmental disabilities; the desire to marry; child bearing and rearing; genetics; appropriate expressions of sexuality; sexual victimization; and unintended pregnancy. Providing participants with factual information related to these issues after discussing sexual attitudes and beliefs relative to individuals with disabilities empowers service providers and increases their levels of comfort and competence. Although it will not be possible to answer all the questions or address all the concerns of participants, providing trainees with skills and incentives to locate their own resources and materials is important. Attending to the affective responses of participants is always a continual and important task of the trainer.

PREPARING PARTICIPANTS FOR INTERVENTIONS

As has been suggested previously, people with disabilities often look to social workers and other helping professionals for information and guidance related to their sexual concerns. To be capable of fulfilling these expectations, social workers must have adequate practice skills to offer basic sexuality education and guidance to their clientele. The third and final portion of a staff training program is devoted to improving the ability of professionals to translate their heightened sensitivity and their increased command of basic facts related to sexuality and to sexuality and disability into the ability to provide concrete services to clients.

The PLISSIT Model (Annon, 1974) will be highlighted, PLISSIT is an acronym which stands for *Permission, Limited Information, Specific Suggestion and Intensive Therapy*. This model was not specifically developed for use with people with disabilities; however, it offers professionals a framework which is particularly useful. Based on a behavioral approach to the treatment of sexual problems, the PLISSIT Model has several strengths. First, it is useful in a variety of settings and can be adapted to whatever treatment time is available. Each ascending level of the PLISSIT Model requires a greater degree of skill, knowledge and training on the part of the social worker. Therefore, practitioners can make decisions about how deeply they want or are able to get involved in the sexual concerns of clients. Having a thorough understanding of the PLISSIT Model can help participants clarify their level of expertise on the four level framework. As social workers reach their limits in terms of level of comfort and competency, appropriate referrals can be made. The facilitator encourages this process by presenting PLISSIT and having participants determine their comfort and skills at each level.

All professionals should be able to provide *Permission* to clients seeking assistance with sexual issues. Permission is offered through statements which provide reassurance to the client that they are not alone or deviant, that their questions or concerns are legitimate and important. Statements of permission are also invitations to clients that the practitioner is available to listen. Permission-type statements should help to create a more relaxed therapeutic atmosphere. Examples of permission-giving statements in response to sexual concerns include:

- You may have questions about how your disability will affect you sexually. If so, I will be happy to discuss them with you.
- That's interesting–tell me more.
- Many women have similar concerns. Let's talk about it.
- I'm glad you brought that up. I can see that it's really important to you.
- Many men are worried about the same thing. Tell me more about what your particular worries are.

A professional effectively opens the door to continued discussion of sexual matters by using permission giving statements. If the helper can do no more than listen and affirm the concerns of the client by offering permission, he or she will have done a great deal. This early discussion is the first step toward clarifying and finding answers to client questions and concerns. Referral is called for if the professional finds that he or she cannot offer any further assistance related to these issues.

Limited Information is the second level of the PLISSIT Model. The practitioner offers the client information related directly to the issue raised in counseling. It is an opportunity to dispel myths and provide brief, factual explanations. Examples of limited information social workers can provide clients include basic explanations of male and female anatomy, discussions of the effects of spinal cord injury on fertility, or the effects of medications on sexual interest. Provision of limited information may include the use of visual materials in addition to verbal explanations. Often, this information will be enough to satisfy the concerns and questions of clients. Limited information is always used in conjunction with an atmosphere of permission. The social worker must possess accurate information to offer clients and staff training sessions are an excellent vehicle for social workers to gain this information. When the information sought exceeds the social worker's expertise, he or she should make a referral to another professional who can provide further assistance.

The next level of the PLISSIT Model, *Specific Suggestions*, necessitates taking a basic sexual history. The social worker can gain a better understanding of the client's ideas and views about any difficulties or concerns and what the individual has previously done to solve any problems. It is also necessary to determine what the client's goals are to ameliorate the sexual problem and to intervene to help meet those goals. For example, in counseling a person with arthritis, the social worker may discover that an individual would like to learn ways to have sexual relationships that are without pain. The practitioner may brainstorm with the client and eventually suggest selecting a specific time in the day when pain medication is most effective, or sexual positions that do not put pressure on painful joints during lovemaking. A specific suggestion for a person with a mobility impairment might include the use of pillows or other supports. Suggesting and facilitating couple's communication is another important strategy. At this level of intervention the social worker will devote considerable time and energy to emotional and psychological needs of the client. This demands more counseling skills and greater sexual knowledge than the more basic levels. If the social worker for any reason does not feel able to provide suggestions, a referral is appropriate.

Intensive Therapy, the fourth level of the model, requires significant skills and knowledge on the part of the professional. Many social workers and counselors may not feel that they can offer

intensive therapy for sexual problems and the training discussed in
this paper is not intended to provide trainees with this level of
expertise. A full sexual history is required as are specialized treatment skills. When clients present with sexual problems requiring
intensive therapy, most social workers will refer these clients to a
specialist.

The PLISSIT Model combines education, guidance, and counseling in a structure that is useful by all levels of professionals. Annon's book provides extensive descriptions and case examples related to the use of this important therapeutic tool.

IMPLEMENTATION OF TRAINING

The successful outcome of staff training is dependent on the
skills and knowledge of the individual who plans and facilitates the
program. Facilities have two choices in this regard: to ask for lead-
ership from a person within the facility or to seek an outside consul-
tant/trainer who can provide the training. Some facilities may be
able to utilize staff who have demonstrated an interest in sexuality
and disability. They may have attended a Sexual Attitude Reassessment workshop or other training, or engaged in independent study
or research. Ideally, these individuals also have the training skills
necessary to develop and facilitate programs for other professionals
or be willing to develop these skills. Facilities using internal staff to
provide staff sexuality training may need to commit resources to
allow potential trainers to gain additional knowledge and develop
skills necessary to develop quality programming. Administrative
support is critical to developing a successful program.

If a staff member is not available to provide sexuality training, an
outside consultant should be considered. There are some advan-
tages to using a consultant. Generally, consultants have developed
basic programs and have relevant materials prepared in advance. A
skilled consultant will add to this basic package, information and
issues specific to the facility or agency. When seeking the services
of a consultant to provide staff training, it is critical that the consultant be knowledgeable in both sexuality and sexuality and disability
and adapt materials to the specific needs of the participant group. It

may be relatively easy to find a trainer to provide a basic desensitization and education program related to general sexuality issues that would be interesting and enjoyable to most staff. However, unless the individual has specific skills and experience working with persons with disabilities, training would most likely be inadequate to prepare participants to work effectively with clients concerned with sexuality and disability. The Coalition on Sexuality and Disability, Inc. in New York City can assist agencies with referrals to skilled training professionals.

Some facilities may choose to invest in the development of one or two staff members who become "resident experts" in sexuality and disability. To increase their expertise, these "experts" could be provided with the time and administrative support to do internships with specialists in sexuality and disability or to do independent study or research. While conferences and workshops devoted specifically to sexuality and disability no longer occur as frequently as they once did, it is important for staff to have the opportunity to attend these programs when possible. Organizations including The Coalition on Sexuality and Disability, Inc., The American Association of Sex Educators, Counselors and Therapists and The Sex Information and Education Council of the United States provide workshops and other training opportunities related to sexuality and sexuality and disability. Local affiliates of Planned Parenthood commonly provide high quality workshops focusing on issues of sexuality and developmental disability.

Regardless of who provides training, it is essential that they receive administrative support. It is less likely that staff will benefit as fully from this opportunity if facility administration does not demonstrate full support and enthusiasm. Training and education takes time and commitment. Staff who are assigned to participate in the training must be allocated the time and be given adequate notice so that training is given a high priority.

Should all staff be required to attend the training? If attendance is left to the discretion of each staff member, those with the greatest need often do not attend the training sessions. Those who readily choose to attend are often rather enlightened and reasonably comfortable already. A well designed program, facilitated by a skilled, sensitive, trainer can provide a non-threatening, educational experience for all who attend–even those who do so with some trepidation or resistance. The experience of simply attending training even as a passive participant may prove valuable.

CONCLUSIONS

It is truly in the best interests of all concerned to provide staff training opportunities related to sexuality and disability. Clients seeking social work services will appreciate the opportunity to receive sexuality related services. For many with disabilities, this will be the first opportunity they have had to deal with very personal sexual issues. For some individuals, an unsuccessful first attempt at acquiring sexual information and guidance may mean that they never try again. Clients will appreciate the fact that sexuality is considered an issue which is important. Spouses and significant others will benefit from sexuality counseling; the quality of sexual relationships will have opportunities to improve or be enhanced as a result of this counseling. It is also important that individuals be offered the opportunity for individual and couple counseling if they so choose.

With training and practice, social workers will grow more comfortable with the sexual and social issues confronted by individuals with disabilities and their spouses/significant others. They will begin to understand that sexuality is an integral part of everyone's life. Having the opportunity to discuss attitudes, values and beliefs, to learn basic factual information related to sexuality and sexuality and disability and to learn a model of sexuality counseling should result in increased feelings of competence for the participants. This comfort should contribute to the creation of a therapeutic environment in which sexuality and sexual issues can be offered the same degree of care and concern as are any other psychosocial issues which individuals with disabilities confront.

The field of sexuality and disability is continually evolving. It is significantly easier in 1993 to access information and audiovisual materials than it was in the 1970s when these issues were first raised. While this is true, several issues still require attention. Sexuality and disability have become a legitimate and important field of study. There is a small group of professionals around the country who have made sexuality counseling and education for individuals with disabilities their specialty. Given that the number of these specialists is limited, there is a great need for social workers to obtain knowledge and develop skills to help people with disabilities and their significant others develop satisfying sexual self images and sexual lives. They can use that knowledge to train other professionals and to directly intervene with clients. These front line professionals are the best defense against the possibility of sexuality and social issues becoming lost in the sometimes overwhelming rehabilitation and human service systems.

REFERENCES

Annon, J. (1974). *The behavioral treatment of sexual problems.* Honolulu: Enabling Systems.

Brashear, D. (1978). Integrating human sexuality into rehabilitation practice. *Sexuality and Disability,* 190-199.

Chipouras, S. (1979). Ten sexuality programs for spinal cord injured persons. *Sexuality and Disability,* 2, 301-321.

Chipouras, S., Cornelius, D., Daniels, S., & Makas, E. (1979). *Who cares? A handbook on sex education and counseling services for disabled people.* Washington, D.C.: George Washington University.

Chubon, R. (1981). Development and evaluation of a sexuality and disability course for the helping professions. *Sexuality and Disability,* 4, 3-14.

Comfort, A. (1978). *Sexual consequences of disability.* Philadelphia, PA: George F. Stickley Company.

Francouer, R. (1991). *Becoming a sexual person.* New York: Macmillan Publishing Company.

Goldsmith, L. (1979). Sexuality and the physically disabled: The work role. *Sexuality and Disability.* 2, 33-37.

Haavik, S., & Menninger, K. (1981). *Sexuality, law and the developmentally disabled person: Legal and clinical aspects of marriage, parenthood and sterilization.* Baltimore: Paul H. Brookes Publishing Company.

Hartman, C., Quinn, J., & Young, B. (1981). *Sexual expression: A manual for trainers.* New York: Human Sciences Press.

Kempton, W. (1987). *Sex education for persons with disabilities that hinder learning: A teacher's guide.* Media, PA: The Amity Road Press.

Monat, R. (1982). *Sexuality and the mentally retarded: A clinical and therapeutic guidebook.* San Diego: College-Hill Press.

Morrison, E., & Underhill Price, M. (1974). *Values in sexuality: A new approach to sex education.* New York: A & W Visual Library.

62 SEXUALITY AND DISABILITIES

Neistadt, M., & Freda, M. (1987). *Choices: A guide to sex counseling with physically disabled adults.* Malabar, FL: Robert E. Krieger Publishing Company.
Rabin, B. (1980). *The sensuous wheeler: Sexual adjustment for the spinal cord injured.* San Francisco: Multi Media Resource Center.
Sandowski, C. (1989). *Sexual concerns when illness or disability strikes.* Springfield, IL: Charles C Thomas.
Schover, L., & Jensen S. (1988). *Sexuality and chronic illness: A comprehensive approach.* New York: The Guilford Press.
Simon, S., Howe, L., & Kirschenbaum, H. (1972). *Values clarification: A handbook of practical strategies for teachers and students.* New York: Hart Publishing Company.
Valois, R., & Kammerman, S. (1984). *Your sexuality: A personal inventory.* New York: Random House.

A Holistic Social Work Approach to Providing Sexuality Education and Counseling for Persons with Severe Disabilities

Romel W Mackelprang

SUMMARY. Spinal cord injuries and other acquired severe neurological disabilities of the spinal cord and peripheral nervous systems can be devastating to people who experience them. People experience changes in mobility and in bowel and bladder function. Sensory, tactile losses are common and physical independence may be compromised. Protracted hospitalizations and rehabilitation may be necessary to develop or regain physical skills and maximize independence. An extremely important, but often neglected, aspect of any comprehensive approach in the rehabilitation of persons affected by severe neurological disabilities is sexual education and counseling. As with any rehabilitation concern, a sexuality program should be approached in a systematic and comprehensive manner. This paper describes one such approach. Originally developed for persons with spinal cord injuries, this approach has been expanded to serve persons with other severe non-cognitive physical disabilities.

Each year, tens of thousands of people in the United States experience neurological disabilities that dramatically and permanently alter their lives. Volitional bowel and bladder control are commonly lost as are sensation and muscle control below injury. Wheelchairs may substitute for legs in everyday mobility. For people with injuries high in the spinal cord, especially those with quadriplegia, respiratory function is compromised and physical independence is diminished (Bedbrook, 1981; Brooks, 1984). People with quadriplegia experience decreased or lost upper extremity function; thus they may need assistance dressing, bathing, and with personal hygiene. During initial hospitalization and rehabilitation, tremendous amounts of time and resources are invested to help people survive once they are discharged.

In the rush to teach and train people to physically "survive," with therapies and treatments lasting several hours each day, medical and allied health professionals sometimes neglect their responsibility to attend to people's psychosocial concerns; those needs that help them to "live." Social workers are often the professionals best equipped to assist clients with emotional coping, adjustments in marital and family relationships and social changes. Psychosocial consequences of disability can have as great an impact on the individual as the physical changes wrought by the disability (Mackelprang, 1986; Trieschmann, 1988).

Although extremely important to most persons with neurological disabilities, sexual adjustment is frequently ignored by health care providers, including social workers. Almost two-thirds are injured between the ages of 15 and 29 (Young, Burns, Bowen, & McCutchen, 1982) when physical sexual development and sexual self image are of paramount concern (Mackelprang & Hepworth, 1990). Disabilities such as spina bifida and muscular dystrophy are lifelong, while others such as multiple sclerosis may originate at any time throughout the life span. The nature and time that a disability occurs in the life cycle are important considerations. Persons in their middle and older adult years have already developed pre-injury sexual self images. They may need assistance adjusting to the many sexual changes severe disability brings. Persons born with disabilities or who experience them in childhood, however, may have a limited sense of their sexuality. Assistance may more appropriately take the form of education on basic sexuality and relationship building.

To provide education and counseling for persons with severe disabilities, it is important for social workers to possess individual, couple and group counseling skills. In addition, extensive knowledge and skills relative to sexuality and sexual adjustment are required. Further, expertise germane to the specific conditions of the people with whom they work is necessary. For example, in working with a young man with paraplegia, the social worker will need to know the neurological mechanisms by which psychogenic and re-flexogenic erections occur and how the lesion affects these nerve pathways. With this knowledge and requisite counseling skills, the social worker is prepared to educate and counsel the client about the erectile implications of his injury. Similarly, when counseling a woman with multiple sclerosis, the social worker may want to address the effects of medications on her spasticity as adductor spasticity in the legs may inhibit the ability to have sexual intercourse.

With these and other severe disabilities, the sexual concerns of clients vary widely. Therefore, it is incumbent upon the social worker to develop organized strategies that are comprehensive enough to address the sexuality concerns of people in general and specific enough to help individuals and couples adjust to the specific illness or disability with which they are faced. In hospitals and rehabilitation centers with high patient volumes, much of the education and counseling can be done in groups designed for patients and partners, with supplemental counseling for individuals and couples. The author has found that, when patient numbers allow, addressing sexual concerns in groups normalizes these issues as participants see that their concerns are shared by others. Groups provide a forum for peer support as people grapple with psychosexual adjustment. Individual and couple's counseling complements education and helps clients with personal sexual questions and problems. It may also be beneficial to invite people who have successfully adjusted to disability (and their partners) to participate, by answering questions and acting as models of people who have adjusted satisfactorily.

This paper describes a model for meeting the education and counseling needs of persons with severe disabilities and their significant others. It is designed to help people develop positive self-images and satisfying sexual lives and consists of five components: (1) Male and female sexual anatomy and physiology are discussed to provide participants with basic understanding of sexual functioning. (2) Disability specific education and counseling are provided to help people understand the general physical implications of their disabilities and how those changes affect their sexual functioning. (3) The sexual-emotional aspects of disability are discussed. With so much emphasis in our society on physical abilities and cosmetic looks, the emotional aspects of sexuality and sexual relationships are ignored in deference to sexual prowess. Therefore, this model highlights the emotional aspects of sexual expression in contrast to a more common performance oriented focus. (4) The physical changes wrought by disability are discussed in terms of the practical implications and sexual options for lovemaking. Neurological disabilities often require people to take actions to avoid problems such as bowel and bladder accidents. In addition, people may be required to modify their methods of sexual expression. (5) Strategies for enhancing sexual self awareness and for beginning or reinitiating sexual contact are provided as people often need specific suggestions to begin the process of positive sexual adjustment.

Originally, the program was developed in a rehabilitation center for persons with acute spinal cord injuries, but the structure is applicable to and has been used for persons with other disabilities and illness. The program provides salient educational information for clients along with counseling for individuals and couples relative to disability for personal concerns that often arise concurrent with education.

MALE AND FEMALE SEXUAL ANATOMY AND PHYSIOLOGY

Explanations of sexual anatomy and the physiology of sexual response are essential components of any sexuality program. Social workers must never assume that clients understand men's and women's sexual anatomy. Slides or pictures depicting internal and external male and female genitalia can be extremely valuable in presenting this material. The social worker can show and describe slides, using them to generate questions and to assess client knowledge. Frank, open discussion models a willingness to talk about sexuality, can help people develop adequate sexual understanding and vocabulary and desensitize clients to sexual conversations.

The social worker, when educating about female sexual anatomy shows and explains each physical structure. These are briefly outlined below. For women, the *vulva* is the region of the external sex organs consisting of the mons veneris, clitoris, labia majora, labia minora and perineum. The *mons veneris* is the area of soft fatty tissue over the pubic bone with numerous sensory nerves that make sexual touch pleasurable and in adults, is covered with hair. The *labia majora* (outer lips) lie close together over the vagina, extending from the mons veneris to the perineum. The *labia minora* (inner lips) are thin folds of tissue which protect the urethral and vaginal openings. Normally closed over the vagina, during sexual arousal they engorge with blood and spread apart to allow vaginal penetration. The *clitoris* is a small sexual organ at the anterior part of the vulva. Homologous to the male penis, it has the same number of nerve endings as the penis and is extremely sensitive to touch. It is unique in that it's only purpose is for sexual pleasure. When women become intensely sexually aroused, the clitoris often retracts protectively under the *clitoral hood*, which normally sits above the clitoris. The *urethral meatus* which lies between the clitoris and vagina is the opening from the bladder and through the urethra for the excretion of urine. The *vagina* lies between the rectum and urethra and is a muscular tubular organ approximately four inches long but which lengthens and widens during sexual arousal and intercourse. It acts as a passageway to the uterus and is the passageway for childbirth and through which menses flow. The *Bartholin's glands* lie near the opening of the vagina and secrete lubricating fluid during sexual arousal. The *uterus* (womb) is a hollow muscular organ about the size and shape of a pear to which a fertilized egg attaches and in which fetus grows. The lining builds up vascular tissue which is expelled during menstruation when a woman is not pregnant. The *cervix* is the narrow, lower end of the uterus which extends into the top of the vagina and through which sperm and menstrual flow pass, and which dilates, allowing a child to pass during childbirth. The *ovaries* are two almond shaped organs on each side of the uterus that secrete female hormones and from which, from puberty to menopause, mature eggs are expelled into neighboring fallopian tubes. The *fallopian tubes* carry eggs that, when fertilized, implant into the uterus.

Male sexual anatomical structures include the *penis* which contains the *urethra* through which urine and semen pass. It contains spongy tissues that engorge when blood flow to the penis increases, causing erections. The head or glans of the penis is very sensitive to touch. At birth the glans is covered by tissue called the foreskin (which is sometimes removed by a process called circumcision). The *scrotum* is a small external pouch containing the testes and that reflexively raises and lowers in response to stimuli such as sexual arousal and temperature changes. The *testes* are contained within the scrotum and produce sperm and male hormones. On the back of each testicle is an *epididymis* which is a tightly wound cord-like structure in which sperm is stored and matured. The *vas deferens* are muscular tubes that carry and propel sperm from the epididymides during ejaculation. As sperm travel along the vas, the *seminal vesicles*, which lie posterior to the bladder, secrete fluid mixing it with the sperm. The fluid has two functions, to provide fructose to give the sperm a source of energy and mobilization and to provide an alkaline environment which neutralizes the acids in the male urethra and the vagina which would otherwise be lethal to sperm. The vas deferens come together at the *prostatic urethra* which functions as a passageway for both urine from the bladder and semen. The *prostate gland* surrounds the prostatic urethra adding fluid which is similar to fluid from the seminal vesicles. This fluid seems to precipitate motility of the sperm which previously has been immobile. The *Cowper's glands* are two pea size glands below the prostate that secrete a few drops of fluid during sexual arousal prior to ejaculation. This fluid neutralizes urine acidity within the urethra prior to ejaculation.

In addition to providing information about sexual anatomy, social workers then discuss sexual response. Masters, Johnson and Kolodny (1985) have conceptualized emotional and physical sexual response into four stages which are very briefly discussed below. The first stage, *excitement*, produces increases in blood pressure, pulse rate and muscle tension. Vasocongestion in the pelvic area increases producing erections in men and vaginal lubrication and swelling of the vulva in women. All these changes are accompanied by psychosexual excitement. The second stage, *plateau*, is characterized by heightened sexual arousal that, with continued stimulation, usually results in orgasm. During plateau, blood pressure, respiration, and pulse rate continue to increase. The scrotum elevates and testes rotate forward in men, while in women, the vagina lengthens, the uterus elevates, and the outer third of the vagina becomes so engorged with blood it narrows. During *orgasm*, which lasts three to ten seconds, rhythmic pelvic contractions occur creating extremely pleasurable sensations and, in men, producing ejaculation. *Resolution* is the stage in which the body returns to its pre-arousal state. Though sexual stimulation has ceased, this stage can be extremely important emotionally and for the relationships of sexual partners.

Comprehensive discussions of sexual anatomy, physiology and sexual response are critical to any educational program to assist people with sexual adjustment. This information is valuable to all, but is especially important to persons with disabilities who may experience alterations in physical response capabilities. The need for comprehensive education is illustrated in the following example from the author's clinical experiences:

> While conducting an educational-counseling group for persons acutely affected by physical disabilities and their partners, Tom, a 27 year old man who had experienced a spinal cord injury several years earlier requested permission to attend. Though his initial rehabilitation had been in a major spinal cord injury center, he related that he had received no sexuality education or counseling. After the first session in which anatomy and physiology were discussed, the man expressed, in an individual session, his surprise that a woman's clitoris is external to the body, having assumed the clitoris is inside the vagina. Post-injury medical procedures had negated his ability to have erections and with limited arm and hand function, he assumed he would never be able to "pleasure a woman sexually." This man's lack of information, combined with several misconceptions had led to a seriously limited lifestyle. After participating in the program, he expressed new found hope that intimate, sexual relationships might be possible for him. Not surprisingly, within three months, he began a relationship with a woman whom he subsequently married.

CONDITION SPECIFIC EDUCATION AND COUNSELING

With an understanding of basic sexual anatomy and physiology, persons with disabilities are better equipped to learn about the sexual changes and implications of disability in their lives. Each disability type or cluster requires specific educational objectives be developed. Counseling needs may also vary depending on the specific effects of the disability for each person.

For persons with severe neurological disabilities such as multiple sclerosis, neuropathy secondary to diabetes, and spinal cord injury, discussion of the central and peripheral nervous systems are critical. For example, basic discussion of sensory and motor pathways in the brain and spinal cord is critical. Issues in client education include explaining normal neurological function in which messages between the brain and the body pass unimpeded through the spinal cord with the brain acting as the master control center of the body. In addition, discussion of the reflex arc, in which the spinal cord operates independently of the brain, is important. An example of this independent function is the well known "knee jerk" reflex that physicians often check by tapping the tendon immediately below the knee cap. This sends sensory messages into the spinal cord that (in addition to traveling to the brain) connect directly to motor neurons leaving the spinal cord causing the thigh muscle to contract and the leg to jerk slightly. Other key areas of education for persons with neurological disabilities include flaccid and spastic areas of injury, cardiovascular function and the relationship between psychological and physical stimulation when sensation is impaired or absent.

Conditions other than neurological disabilities require different educational foci. Concerns to be addressed for people with cardiovascular disabilities, for example, include a basic understanding of the heart and circulatory system, the effects of medications on the sympathetic and parasympathetic nervous systems that affect heart rate and blood pressure, and influences of different types of exercise. Persons with chronic pain will benefit from comprehensive explanations of factors that influence pain perception and strategies to ameliorate pain.

Spinal cord injuries pose another set of educational and counseling issues. For men with spinal cord injuries, knowledge of reflex arc can be utilized to understand mechanisms by which erections occur. Reflexogenic erections, which are controlled at the sacral (lowest) levels of the spinal cord are possible for many men with spinal cord injuries because, if the nerves in the sacral region of the spinal cord are not directly injured, they continue to function independent of brain input. Thus, in a way similar to the "knee jerk" reflex, proper genital stimulation can produce reflex erections for spinal cord injured men, even when genital sensation is absent.

Psychogenic erections, on the other hand, are most often lacking in men with serious damage to the spinal cord. The social worker can help clients understand that psychogenic erections occur when messages from the sexual centers of the brain descend through the spinal cord exiting in the low thoracic, high lumbar section of the spinal cord. The combination of this mental stimulation and activation of nerves in the sacral regions of the spinal cord produce psychogenic erections in response to sexual arousal. When input from the brain is interrupted in the spinal cord or peripheral nervous systems, psychogenic erection capability is adversely affected. Thus most men with spinal cord injuries lose psychogenic erection capabilities.

Other critical issues to be addressed include ejaculation and fertility which in men with spinal cord injuries are seriously affected. Infertility treatment methods such as intrathecal neostigmine injection, subcutaneous physostigmine injection, and electroejaculation techniques (Sipski and Alexander, 1991a) should be discussed as should the limited success rates of these infertility treatments.

Women with spinal cord injuries also have concerns (Sipski and Alexander, 1991b) that can be addressed once general knowledge of their disability has been established. Unlike men, women's spinal cord function has little effect on reproductive capacity, however, women have many other concerns. For example, women with acute spinal cord injury often experience temporary amenorrhea. Before resuming sexual activity, they need to be informed that menstrual disruption does not signal infertility. The need for prompt intervention in this area is illustrated below:

Jeri was a 22 year old newlywed woman with an acute spinal cord injury. As part of her rehabilitation program, she was granted a weekend home pass six weeks after her injury. Having received no sexuality education or counseling prior to her home visit, she assumed that since she missed two menstrual periods, she did not have to worry about birth control, therefore, she and her husband resumed sexual intercourse without using contraceptives. Only after talking with a nurse about her sexual experiences was she alerted to the possibility of becoming pregnant. Fortunately, Jeri did not become pregnant, but experienced significant stress while waiting to see if she was pregnant, to the extent of threatening legal action against her health care providers for not educating her properly.

Social workers can be key in providing education about contraceptive options available to women with spinal cord injuries and similar disabilities by informing them about the implications of their disabilities, then applying the implications to sexual and contraceptive matters. For example, oral contraceptives may be contraindicated because of the increased incidence of blood clots in the legs when people are neurologically impaired. Lack of abdominal sensation is a contraindication for IUDs. For women with higher level injuries, manual dexterity may be diminished, influencing the ability to use such contraceptive devices as foam, cervical caps, and diaphragms. Condoms are often the contraceptive of choice for women with spinal cord injury (Sipski, & Alexander, 1991b) and social workers will want to discuss all the options and implications of each method of contraception.

With a proper foundation of disability specific knowledge, people will be better prepared to apply their understanding to the specific sexual implications of their disabilities. They will have an increased understanding of their disabilities and be prepared to make informed choices. By educating persons about the general physical and sexual implications specific to their disabilities, social workers empower them to become experts about their own bodies, to be able to make sexual decisions and to solve problems they face. The value of disability specific education is illustrated in the following case:

Frank was a 32 year old man with spina bifida who sought counseling with the author. His parents and health care providers had never discussed sexuality or given him messages that he was a sexual person as he grew up (especially since, when he was born, the life expectancy for persons with spina bifida was short). He had taken a human sexuality course in college, but prior to receiving counseling, he had no idea what his sexual capabilities were. He was invited to participate in a sexuality group for people with neurological disabilities. From the group, he gained knowledge about the effects of neurological damage on sexual function. Since spina bifida results from a neurological defect, he generalized the information provided in group to understand the specific effects of his spina bifida. He reported that the group experience was the first time in his life that someone had explained the reasons his body functioned as it did. His sexual understanding provided him the confidence to begin exploring relationships with women and he soon began dating.

An example of the value of disability specific education and counseling irrespective of age is illustrated by another case example:

Mr. Wight, age 81 and his 83 year old wife, approached the author for counseling prior to Mr. Wight's home visit from a rehabilitation center four weeks after a stroke. The Wights' had enjoyed a physically intimate relationship prior to Mr. Wight's stroke but were worried that sexual contact would precipitate another stroke. They were relieved to find that his activity levels in therapy approximated levels engaged in during sexual contact. Information was provided about blood pressure and heart rate during various activities including sex. The couple was provided general information about Mr. Wight's stroke that was then applied to their sexual lives. In a subsequent meeting, the couple reported that their weekend visit went well emotionally and sexually. Sexual fears were ameliorated and problems prevented. Subsequent sexual counseling was provided to deal with additional concerns as they arose.

With an understanding of the biological and physical implications of their conditions, persons with disabilities will be better prepared to apply that information specifically to their unique sexual issues and concerns as the social worker counsels with them.

EMOTIONAL ASPECTS OF SEXUALITY
AND DISABILITY

The emotional or psychological impact of disabilities on persons who experience them and on their partners can be profound. In addition to physical sexual concerns, attention to psychosocial adjustment is an essential component of any sexuality program, including attention to body image and self-esteem (Schatzlein, 1991; Mackelprang & Hepworth, 1990).

People with disabilities that result in sensory or mobility impairment may wonder whether or not sex can be pleasurable when genital sensation is lost. Coping with diminished or absent genital sensation is very difficult. The lack of previously erotic tactile sensation may leave people wondering how sexual contact can become pleasurable again (Mackelprang & McDonald, 1988). Lack of mobility may make it impossible to perform sexually in ways they have been accustomed to performing. Atrophied limbs, spasticity, urine bags, and the need for physical assistance can all contribute to low sexual self-image.

Psychosocial intervention is critical as social workers help clients deal with losses and develop new sexual coping strategies. In group discussions and in individual and couple counseling, social workers can help clients begin reframing sexual expectations and perceptions. A common misconception held in society is the idea that the genitals are *the* primary sources of sexual pleasure, often ignoring the emotional and mental aspects of sexuality. Examples can be used to illustrate the importance of the brain in sexuality and sexual pleasure. People can be encouraged to recount experiences they have had in which they read or viewed material that aroused them sexually. They might be asked to relate a time when a personal sexual memory triggered subsequent sexual feelings and arousal. The brain is the source of these responses: excitement occurring in the absence of any physical, genital contact.

Clients with neurological disabilities will experience changes in sensations to varying degrees. For example, people with strokes of the middle cerebral artery usually experience sensory and mobility impairments on one side of the body, while those with spina bifida will have impairment most often in the lower extremities and genitals. It is important for social workers to acknowledge the limitations caused by the disability but also to help clients understand the potentials for pleasure (Mackelprang & Neubauer, 1990). They can teach clients that their entire skin surface is covered with billions of nerve endings that are sensitive to touch and physically pleasurable. Regardless of the type or extent of disability, the neck, ears, and face retain sensation. Depending on the level of impairment, the chest, breasts, and other areas of the body may also retain sensation. Communicating that the entire skin surface of the body, from head to toe, is the largest "sexual organ" may help persons with limitations begin to focus on sexual possibilities rather than just grieving over sexual limitations or losses.

Even though tactile sensation may be impaired for certain areas of the body, social workers can help clients understand the importance of their other senses that can compensate for losses. The senses of sight, hearing, taste and smell have almost limitless possibilities for sexual enjoyment and clients can learn that their sensual experiences will be enhanced when these senses are more fully developed. Clients can also be encouraged to attend to the enjoyment derived from pleasuring their sexual partners as the partners' responses can be incorporated into their own sexual passion.

Orgasms are almost always affected by neurological disabilities. Some people lose orgasmic capability. Others may still retain orgasmic capabilities, but their orgasms may be less genitally and physically focused and more mentally centered than prior to the disability. Though almost always perceived as different from previous orgasms, people still find them enjoyable and satisfying. Even people who do not experience orgasms after disability find sex to be very gratifying. Social workers can help clients understand that lovemaking is a process. Counseling can be used to emphasize that closeness, touching, giving and receiving pleasure can be satisfying for both partners, even in the absence of orgasm. Clients who report orgasmic absence often report a pleasurable prolonged period of warmth with intense sexual contact. Most clients are concerned with orgasm capability and should be informed of the ramifications of their conditions; however, counselors can help clients focus on the process of lovemaking rather than the goal of orgasm.

The emotional and perceptual aspects of sexuality are vital components of client sexuality and among the most important areas of intervention for social workers. People's perceptions of the disability and feelings about themselves and their sexual capabilities are as important as the actual physical implications of their disabilities. Counseling and educational efforts necessarily inform people of their changes and limitations, but equally important is to help them focus efforts on their retained abilities. Helping clients to maintain a positive, though somewhat modified sexual identity is a primary goal of this model.

The importance of attending to emotional concerns is represented in the following example:

Rob was a 24 year old man with a low, incomplete spinal cord injury who sought counseling two months after his injury with Renee, his 25 year old wife of two years. Rob and Renee had attended two educational group sexuality sessions when they met with the author in couple counseling. During their first couple session, Rob stated that he planned to divorce Renee so she could find a "normal husband who will satisfy her sexually." Though his injury was far less severe than other participants in the sexuality group in which he was participating, he felt devastated by his injury and believed he would be doing his wife a favor by divorcing her. His wife, on the other hand, was distraught over Rob's attitude and his rejection of her. Renee repeatedly expressed her desire to be close to her husband physically and emotionally and was devastated when he rejected her attempts at closeness. To help this couple, a combination of group and couple counseling was used. Intervention in group focused on education about sexuality in general and spinal cord injury specifically. In addition, opportunities were provided for group participants to support each other through group discussions. In couple's counseling, the basic needs for closeness and intimacy for both Rob and Renee were discussed and suggestions were provided to enhance their intimacy through physical closeness. Renee was encouraged to express her needs to be emotionally close and her continued physical attraction to him. Similarly, Rob told Renee that his love and caring for her motivated him to seek what he perceived was in her best interest. To assist in couple's counseling, Marian and Will, a couple who had successfully adjusted to Will's spinal cord injury, were invited to attend a counseling session. They spoke frankly and openly of their adjustment processes, provided concrete sexual ideas and suggestions and offered future support if Rob or Renee so desired. One of the most important contributions Marian and Will made was the role modeling they provided. Their adjustment and happiness together helped both Rob and Renee see their own possibilities, making them more open to the social worker's subsequent counseling suggestions. The combination of group and couple counseling, supplemented with support from another couple who had gone through similar experiences helped improve the self-esteem of both Rob and Renee, strengthened their marriage and substantially enhanced their sexual relationship.

Though Rob's disability was the least severe among those participating in sexuality group, Rob and Renee needed more support and intervention than the other participants in their sexuality group because of Rob's negative perceptions of the impact of his disability and the effect his reactions had on their relationship.

PRACTICAL SEXUAL CONCERNS AND SEXUAL OPTIONS

Another component of a sexuality program involving severe neurological disability is attention to the practical aspects of lovemaking. These practical concerns may include issues such as bowel and bladder function, spasticity management, and balancing the roles of caregiver/care-receiver with roles as lovers.

Voluntary bladder function is highly susceptible to impairment when people experience neurological disabilities. When this occurs, a bladder management program is required, often calling for a catheter to empty the bladder. When an indwelling catheter is used, the couple may choose to keep it in place during lovemaking. If so, the catheter should be secured, usually by taping it to the body, to prevent tugging on the catheter that may traumatize the bladder neck or urethral meatus. Suprapubic catheters and ileodiversionary devices should be similarly secured. Men who wear indwelling catheters during intercourse should tape the tubing to the base of the penis and liberally apply water soluble lubricants so the catheter will not cause irritation for the sexual partner. People with impaired bladder control who opt to remove catheters, use intermittent catheterization, or who do not catheterize will want to restrict fluid intake for at least two hours before sexual contact and empty their bladders prior to sexual activity to avoid accidents. In addition, they may want to avoid vigorous abdominal stimulation that may trigger bladder emptying. Almost everyone with loss of bladder control will experience occasional accidents. In addition to addressing the above concerns, counseling can help people to minimize the trauma associated with such accidents during lovemaking. Suggesting that couples keep a towel available and/or incorporate showering into lovemaking activities can help couples cope with accidents should they occur.

Bowel accidents can usually be prevented if people take precautions. For example, people with spinal cord injuries often follow a program in which they evacuate the bowel every two days, through digital stimulation, manual evacuation or by using suppositories. To avoid bowel accidents during lovemaking, the social worker will counsel clients to avoid certain activities. For example, making love prior to a scheduled bowel program is not recommended as abdominal and genital stimulation may trigger a full bowel to move. Lovemaking after a meal may also be unwise as food entering the digestive system triggers digestive peristalsis and, when combined with lovemaking, may trigger a bowel movement. As with the bladder, bowel accidents may occasionally occur; however, as social workers educate and help people become familiar with their bodies, they can take precautions to minimize accidents and cope with accidents when they occur.

The ability to manage the dual roles of caregiver and lover is an extremely important issue that couples face when a disability is severe. When the person with the disability needs help with personal care such as bowel and bladder management and dressing, partners generally provide much of this assistance. Some sexual partners are not bothered by the dual roles of caregiver and lover and may even find satisfaction incorporating caregiving activities such as undressing and bathing into lovemaking. Others may find it is difficult to help with such activities as bowel programs and bladder care, then fill the role of lover as well. Social workers will want to address this issue with couples and, when indicated, assist them to explore options for obtaining physical assistance for personal care such as bowel and bladder programs, dressing and hygiene from outside sources.

Attention to the practical concerns of love making is critical to sexual education and counseling efforts. If these issues are neglected, people may become intimidated and unwilling to risk the embarrassment of accidents during sexual intimacy. The importance of addressing practical concerns of lovemaking is illustrated by the following case:

> Marilyn was a 43 year old woman who used an indwelling catheter because of bladder control problems secondary to severe multiple sclerosis. In addition, she had significant spasticity in her lower extremities. These conditions, combined with Marilyn's motor deficits, intimidated Marilyn and her lover Jamie, and inhibited their sexual intimacy. The social worker suggested to Marilyn that she tape the catheter tubing to her abdomen during sexual contact to prevent it from tugging on and traumatizing her urethra and bladder. As Marilyn's spasticity was exacerbated by genital and abdominal stimulation and inhibited love making, the social worker, together with Marilyn and Jamie, consulted with Marilyn's neurologist, and he agreed to alter Marilyn's medications which ameliorated some of her spasticity.

With bladder and spasticity problems ameliorated, Marilyn and Jamie were better prepared to resume intimate sexual contact that had ceased as Marilyn's multiple sclerosis had become more severe. Another couple benefitted from suggestions in the sexuality group they were attending to combine and incorporate personal hygiene into lovemaking activities:

Art was a 37 year old man with quadriplegia. He required bowel care help which his 35 year old wife, Betty provided. When Betty would do Art's bowel program, she would also help Art shower. As a result of suggestions offered in sexuality group, Betty began to join Art in the shower. Both loved the sensuality of the water and soap and their physical closeness and they would frequently continue lovemaking in bed after showering.

Methods of sexual expression are altered following neurological disability. As previously discussed, sensation and mobility may be diminished or lost, spasticity and hyperreflexia may need monitoring and men may experience erectile and ejaculation loss. It is critical that social workers intervene to help clients begin exploring physical changes in their bodies and to assess their responses to sexual stimulation. They can help couples discuss and reassess methods of expression and determine practices with which they feel comfortable.

Sexual intercourse is an option for many men and almost all women. When a male has a disability that affects erections, couples will benefit from suggestions to identify types of stimulation (such as direct penis contact, pulling thigh hair, or applying heat or cold to the groin area) that precipitate and maintain reflexogenic erections. Regardless of erectile capabilities, it is important to discuss other options such as oral-genital and manual stimulation.

Sexual positioning is often changed following disability. The affected person may lack mobility requiring the non-disabled partner to be more physically active than previously. Because of physical limitations, some former activities may be impossible. Sometimes supports, such as pillows, for affected limbs are useful for positioning. Alternate methods of sexual expression are often desired.

Explicit discussion is critical when the social worker is exploring sexual options with clients. Manual stimulation, using hands, arms, legs, or other body parts is used by many people to provide sexual pleasure. Though used by many persons without disabilities, manual stimulation may become an especially important means of sexual expression for people with disabilities. Oral-genital sex is also discussed. For some people, oral stimulation may be the only means they have of active sexual expression. Some may have never attempted oral sex and are relieved when their fears are ameliorated through open and honest discussion with a social worker. Use of assistive devices such as vibrators is often valuable. Assistive devices may enhance stimulation when there is diminished sensation and assist in partner pleasuring when mobility is limited. The author has found that showing a variety of sexual aids such as vibrators to people in group and couple's sessions can be extremely valuable.

A major concern for many people is the effect diminished or absent sensation has on sexual pleasure. The social worker can help these people learn that areas of the body where sensation remains intact can become heightened centers of pleasure. Touching and caressing areas such as the neck, chest and ears can be extremely pleasurable and more erotic than in the absence of disability. The social worker can also help people explore whether or not touch to areas of the body that lack sensation may be enjoyable. Some people find that seeing and thinking about a partner's touch is pleasurable, even in the absence of tactile sensation.

A major focus of counseling about sexual options is an emphasis on the brain (rather than the genitals) as the primary sex organ. Counselors can emphasize that genital function is not synonymous with sexual function. The extent of sexual pleasure that people experience is largely determined by their attitudes about sex and their willingness to explore new avenues of sexual expression. Critical to these discussions is an emphasis on partner communication. As sex is discussed in counseling, the social worker models openness and desensitizes people, helping them talk openly about sexuality.

The range of sexual experiences varies widely. When discussing sexuality with one man with quadriplegia, the man explained that he was able to have orgasms when his partner touched, caressed and licked his face, neck, and chest. He described his orgasms as more emotionally based than orgasms before his injury, but still extremely pleasurable. Many other persons have reported similar abilities.

As people learn to cope with sexual alterations subsequent to disability, it is essential they begin to develop or reestablish com-munication and relationships with their partners. The person with the disability will be better prepared to discuss the sexual implica-tions of the disability, both limitations and capabilities. Couples may need help discussing wants, likes, dislikes, fears, desires, con-cerns and expectations. As they discuss practical lovemaking con-cerns such as catheters, spasticity, muscle atrophy, and bowel and bladder management, they will be able to circumvent many prob-lems and eliminate surprises. They can also evaluate together, sexu-al activities and preferences. Closeness and intimacy can be fos-tered as they share their feelings and work together to enhance their relationships. Some couples find the increased closeness and under-standing that is developed by enhanced communication compen-sates for physical losses and enhances emotional and physical inti-macy.

Initially, it is difficult for people to discuss or even acknowledge physical changes caused by disability, or they may be embarrassed with the intimate problems they face. They may be afraid they will be unable to perform as they would like. Fear of rejection may inhibit people from talking with partners about sex. Social work counseling can begin the process of couple communication about sexuality as the social worker creates an environment of trust and openness. Initially, people may be nervous, but with a foundation of knowledge provided through sexuality education, couples will be better prepared to take the risk to actively begin sexual relation-ships.

STRATEGIES FOR INITIATING SEXUAL CONTACT

While education and counseling help couples understand sexual-ity and the effects of disability on sexuality and sexual activity, a crucial component of sexuality education and counseling is helping couples apply the knowledge they have received to their respective sexual lives. For some people with disabilities and their partners, this can be very frightening. They may be afraid that they will not be able to perform, will not enjoy sexual contact, will not satisfy their partners or they may be overwhelmed by problems such as catheters or spasticity.

As the social worker helps couples initiate sexual intimacy, three areas of focus are important. First, persons with disabilities will want to find out about or rediscover their bodies. Body self-exploration or masturbation is useful for people to identify sensory areas that lack sensation, other areas that have altered sensations and those regions of the body with intact sensation. Using self exploration, people with sensory alterations become aware of the regions of the body that can take on added sexual significance, for example, the neck, ears and chest. Self exploration is assigned by the social worker in such a way that there is no expectation of heightened sexual arousal, thus removing the fear of failure. As people become more comfortable with their bodies using self exploration, the social worker can increasingly define self exploration in more sexually exploratory terms, encouraging clients to attend to sexual feelings and share their discoveries with their partners. The following case is illustrative of the use of self exploration or masturbation:

Joan was a 21 year old woman with a congenital spinal cord injury and absent genital sensation who, along with her 22 year old fiance Tom, requested premarital sexual counseling. Neither Joan nor Tom had prior sexual experience, and because of moral, religious concerns, they were not comfortable with sexual activity prior to their marriage. The social worker suggested self-exploration to Joan as a way of becoming knowledgeable about those areas of her body that might be pleasurable to sexual touch. Initially Joan expressed reservations about this because of religious prohibitions against masturbation so the social worker consulted, with Joan's consent, with her minister about the value of self-exploration in the context of her situation. As a result, the minister lent his support to self-exploration, reinforced their counseling efforts, and encouraged sexual discussions between Joan and Tom. Joan began to better learn about her body sexually, and with her minister's blessing, shared these discoveries in counseling sessions. Though the couple was not physically intimate prior to their marriage, they discussed physical and practical concerns, sexual options and shared activities they might want to experiment with after their marriage. After four sessions with the social worker, the couple felt sexually prepared enough to deal with sex in their marriage and were married shortly thereafter with the understanding that they seek marital sexual counseling as needed.

For Joan and Tom, Joan's use of premarital self-exploration, combined with frank discussions with Tom, were the primary means of sexually preparing for their sexual relationship.

Self-other pleasuring or sensate focus is an additional strategy that may be recommended for couples as a way to enhance both communication and sexual expression. Couples are instructed to find a place that is private and interruption free. After removing clothing, the partner without a disability begins by touching and caressing the partner with the disability. The "giver" asks for feedback about how specific kinds of touch feel and areas of the body that are pleasurable when caressed. The "receiver" is to give regular feedback and direction to the "giver," guiding the giver in how and where to touch. Areas of the body to be touched include those regions that may lack or have diminished sensation. In addition, practical concerns such as catheter placement can be addressed. After sufficient exploration, the roles then switch; the partner having the disability provides the touch and receives constant feedback. Equal attention is paid to both persons as giver and receiver of pleasure. Self-other pleasuring is extremely important in facilitating partner sexual communication. It facilitates their sexual discussion and learning without expectations that they perform sexually. It reduces the fear so common among persons with disabilities, that they are not sexual beings. Couples gain knowledge about alterations in sensation caused by the disability, and begin developing sexual practices based on their experiences. Often, they find that areas of the body without sensation can still be sources of pleasure as they see and experience the intimacy of their partner's touch. In addition, as the person with the disability acts as "giver," limitations in mobility and in the ability to provide pleasure are identified and couples can learn to compensate for mobility limitations. The social worker can help couples with suggestions, provide support and help with any frustrations they may experience. To prevent performance failure, the social worker sets no expectation that participants will experience sexual arousal orgasm in the early sensate focus sessions.

As couples increasingly feel comfortable together and develop understanding of changes (strengths, potentials, and limitations) brought by disability, the focus of self-other pleasuring becomes more overtly sexual. Couples are encouraged to learn about their sexual pleasures together. Communication is still a primary focus and couples are encouraged to talk all throughout sensate focus sessions. The process of the sexual experience is emphasized and goal oriented, orgasm focused behavior is minimized. Some persons with diminished or absent sensation will eventually experience orgasms while others will not. However, with the focus on sexual process, the need for orgasm becomes secondary or unimportant over time.

As couples become increasingly sexually active, their knowledge and comfort will be enhanced and they will find answers to their questions together. For example, they may find ways to achieve and maintain erections, deal with spasticity, or work around urinary problems. They will develop methods to enhance pleasure, such as through oral and manual stimulation. It is incumbent on the social worker to help couples explore, experiment, and communicate during regular educational and counseling sessions and by giving and following up on homework assignments. Again, the case of Joan and Tom is illustrative:

> Shortly after their marriage, Joan and Tom contacted the social worker for follow up counseling. They reported they were enjoying their physical intimacy, but wanted to enhance their lovemaking. Tom wanted to learn more about how to help Joan feel pleasure and Joan was concerned with Tom's satisfaction. Sensate focus sessions were prescribed. Through this, the couple found that Joan enjoyed experiencing Tom's touching her in the genital region (if she could see the touch) even though she lacked tactile sensation. They also found Joan's sensory band where her sensation began to change from normal was particularly sensitive to touch. Among other things, the couple found they especially enjoyed lying side by side

with the length of their bodies touching as they caressed each other.

The knowledge Joan and Tom gained was developed over the course of several sessions. They would engage in sensate focus sessions, talk about their experiences privately afterwards and would further process their experiences in counseling sessions with the social worker. The social worker would, in turn, provide feedback and offer suggestions for future sensate focus sessions. Joan and Tom found that their intimacy was enhanced as they slowly, and without performance expectations, grew and learned together.

CONCLUSIONS

Social workers working with persons who have disabilities have a responsibility to help clients cope with the many psychosocial concerns they face. An important, but often ignored aspect of adjustment is sexuality and sexual functioning. When developing a sexual education and counseling program, it is important to identify the needs of individual clients and client groups, and develop programs that systematically and comprehensively address these needs. This paper outlines one approach used successfully with persons with neurological disabilities such as multiple sclerosis and spinal cord injury. Included in the program are specific content areas on: (a) sexual anatomy, (b) physiology of the sexual response, (c) condition specific education and counseling, (d) emotional concerns affecting client sexuality, (e) practical physical sexual knowledge, (f) sexual options, and (g) sexual relationships. A comprehensive program can be provided through individual and couple's counseling. When there are sufficient numbers of participants, group education and counseling can complement individual and couple's counseling. Programs addressing the concerns of clients with other disabilities should be developed to address their specific disabilities and counseling of individuals and couples should be personalized.

The emphasis social work places on holistic intervention on behalf of clients along with an empowerment oriented intervention strategy, uniquely prepares social workers to help clients with disabilities and their partners cope with the many psychosocial changes that accompany disabilities. Social workers who are prepared with counseling skills and disability specific sexual knowledge can have a major influence on positive psychosexual development and adjustment of clients with disabilities and their partners. It is up to the profession and up to individual social workers to meet this important need.

REFERENCES

Bedbrook, G. (1981). *The care and management of spinal cord injuries.* New York: Springer Verlag New York Inc.

Brooks, N.A. (1984). From rehabilitation to independent living. In A.P. Ruskin (Ed.), *Current therapy in physiatry: Physical medicine and rehabilitation* (pp. 536-548). Philadelphia: W.B. Saunders.

Mackelprang, R.W. (1986). Social and emotional adjustment following spinal cord injury. Salt Lake City: Unpublished doctoral dissertation.

Mackelprang, R.W. & Neubauer, R.L. (1990). Sexuality and sexual adjustment after stroke: Implications for social work. *Arete, 15* (2), 1-10.

Mackelprang, R.W. & Hepworth, D.L. (1990). Sexual adjustment following spinal cord injury: Empirical findings and clinical implications. *Arete, 15* (1) 1-13.

Mackelprang, R.W. & McDonald, B.B. (1988). *A guide to sexuality following spinal cord injury.* Salt Lake City: University of Utah.

Masters, W.H., Johnson, V.E. & Kolodny, R.C. (1985). Human sexuality (2nd ed.). Boston: Little, Brown & Company.

Schatzlein, J. (1991). Body image/self-esteem: A time for focus and control. *SCI Psychosocial Process, 4* (2), 41-44.

Sipski, M.L. & Alexander, C.J. (1991a). Infertility following spinal cord injury: Current methods of treatment. *SCI Psychosocial Process, 4* (2), 45-48.

Sipski, M.L. & Alexander, C.J. (1991b). Female sexuality following spinal cord injury. *SCI Psychosocial Process, 4* (2), 49-52.

Trieschmann, R.B. (1988). *Spinal cord injuries: Psychological, social, and vocational rehabilitation.* New York: Pergamon Press Inc.

Young, J.S., Burns, P.E., Bowen, A.M. & McCutchen, R. (1982). *Spinal cord injury statistics: Experience of the regional spinal cord injury systems.* Phoenix: Good Samaritan Medical Center.

Cognitive Impairments:
Psychosocial and Sexual Implications
and Strategies
for Social Work Intervention

Gary Sigler
Romel W Mackelprang

SUMMARY. Cognitive impairments, including learning disability, traumatic brain injury, and minimal brain dysfunction, have characteristics that include impulsiveness, communication skill deficits, difficulties with reasoning and problem solving, and impaired self-concept. Without professional intervention, these problems are likely to lead to marginal social acceptance, low levels of intimacy, and impaired sexuality development. This paper describes selected cognitive and behavioral implications of cognitive impairments and the influences of cognitive impairments on sexuality. Suggestions for social work interventions are provided to help persons with cognitive impairments develop positive self-images and values, and to help them establish satisfying intimate and sexual relationships.

Cognitive impairments (CI) are a group of related disabilities that are widespread in our society. Though the causes of CI vary, and include traumatic brain injury (TBI), learning disabilities, and minimal brain dysfunction (MBD), many of the resulting needs and limitations of persons affected by CI are similar. For example, memory disorders and impulsiveness are common characteristics of CI (Ceci, Ringstorm & Lea, 1981; Torgesen, 1984) and treatment modalities, based on individual needs are similar, regardless of the etiology (Prigitano, 1988).

When people are diagnosed with CI, interventions commonly focus on ameliorating problems in academic areas such as reading, writing, language and mathematics. Unfortunately, CI affects life skills such as social interaction, decision making, interpersonal problem solving, judgment and sexuality; however, human services professionals often leave these problems untreated. Thus, persons with CI may be taught to read and solve mathematical equations but not helped to develop the skills that are critical for social acceptance and group membership even though people with CI themselves identify social interaction as more problematic than academic deficits (Pihl & McLarnon, 1984).

A psychosocial consequence of CI that receives scant attention from professionals is sexuality. Unlike conditions such as many physical disabilities for which sexuality concerns may be functional and obvious, the effects of CI on sexuality are more subtle and prone to be neglected. Problems associated with CI often result in low self esteem, distorted self-image and social isolation that adversely affect sexual self-image and the quality of intimate relationships. Thus, while CI does not impair physical sexual functioning, the broad range of thoughts, feelings, and interactions encompassed by sexuality (Mahoney, 1983), are often adversely influenced. This paper, therefore, addresses the psychosocial implications of CI, and the effects of these implications on sexual development and sexuality. Suggestions for social work intervention with persons with CI are also provided.

SELECTED COMMON CHARACTERISTICS OF COGNITIVE IMPAIRMENTS

Though there is substantial heterogeneity among individuals with CI and though individuals vary in the degree their disabilities affect them (Bender, 1992), there are common characteristics. These problems include impulsiveness, reasoning and problem solving, group membership and social acceptance, self-concept, and communication skills and have been selected for presentation in this article because of their pervasiveness and prevalence in individuals with CI.

Impulsiveness

A characteristic common to individuals with CI is impulsiveness (Epstein, Cullinan, & Sternberg, 1977; Lezak & O'Brien, 1990), defined as a reaction to stimuli that is completed quickly and without consideration of consequences (Carbo, 1983). Impulsiveness becomes problematic when individuals exhibit high rates of misjudgment or social inappropriateness (Epstein, Cullinan, & Sternberg, 1977). The following case is illustrative of impulsiveness:

A young man with TBI, Terry, had two months of successful employment when he was asked by his employer to plug an appliance into an electrical outlet. As he did, he pretended to receive a severe electrical shock, frightening, then enraging his co-workers. Terry's act of impulsiveness damaged his social belonging and threatened his continued employment. His vocational rehabilitation counselor referred him for counseling and training to assist him to identify social cues and contexts and to respond with appropriate behaviors after which he returned to employment with the same company. With improved understanding and control of his impulsive behavior, his interpersonal relationships in the company improved and he became accepted as a peer group member.

Terry's impulsiveness resulted in embarrassment, social estrangement, and employment suspension. Only after professional intervention did he comprehend the personal and social consequences of his behavior and more effectively begin to control his impulsiveness.

Problem Solving and Communication Problems

Problem solving difficulties for individuals with CI (unlike persons with mental retardation), are not due to low general intellectual functioning but to the inability to select relevant stimuli from the environment and to associate the stimuli with the current need or action. Their behavior, therefore, may be based on misinterpretations of environmental stimuli. Other times, persons may interpret the stimuli correctly, but their behaviors are inappropriate for the context.

Communication deficits in persons with CI may be pervasive and problematic throughout their lives. Expressive communication deficits may be manifest by an inability to express thoughts in writing or to articulate ideas verbally. Receptive deficits prevent the persons from adequately interpreting information from their environments. Children with communication deficits have difficulty in school, with peers, and at home. In addition, adults with CI have difficulties in vocational settings often resulting in unemployment or underemployment (Blalock & Johnson, 1987).

The following case is illustrative of problems encountered as a result of problem solving and communicative deficits:

> Stephanie, age 29, had a history of vocational failure. She had held numerous jobs for short periods. A common complaint by employers was that she was too slow and required excessive supervision to complete tasks. Though she would receive verbal instructions from supervisors, she was unable to translate these instructions into action, especially in stressful or demanding situations. One job she held was in a fast food restaurant taking and filling orders at the counter. She reported that the work was going well the first day until the noon customer rush when she became confused and overwhelmed with the multiple demands placed on her. Unable to articulate her frustrations to her supervisor and incapable of carrying out multiple demands placed on her, she ran from the restaurant screaming.

In reviewing the situation with Stephanie, it became clear she was unable to problem solve by prioritizing which of the numerous tasks needing her attention were the most important. This was compounded by her receptive communication deficits in which the discrete steps of her supervisors' instructions were not assimilated. Her inability to prioritize tasks left her feeling overwhelmed and she was unable to fulfill her responsibilities adequately. This, in turn, resulted in multiple job failures.

For Stephanie, like others with CI, the difficulty with problem solving is often the result of using inefficient problem solving strategies (Torgesen, Murphy, & Ivey, 1979; Richey & McKinney, 1978). Compounded by the effects of impaired communication skills Stephanie, like others, experienced repeated failures in spite of normal intelligence and high motivation for success.

Social Acceptance and Self Concept

As a result of a combination of factors (including impulsiveness, reasoning difficulties, and communication deficits) persons with CI often experience difficulty with group membership (Kelly, Wildman, Urey, & Thurman, 1979) and peer acceptance. People may not be completely rejected; rather they often remain on the social fringes of group activities and associations (Bender, Bailey, Stuck, & Wyne, 1984). Human development, including the development of adult responsibility, is dependent upon associations with peers and the ability to be a functioning member of one or more social groups. Failure in group membership is detrimental to the development of mature adults.

Self-concept, formed from a person's reactions to the sum of life events, is affected in persons with CI (Horn, O'Donnell, & Vitulano, 1983). Individuals with CI achieve less success than their peers and may not believe they have control over their successes (Gregory, Shanahan, & Walberg, 1986). As a consequence, they are less likely than others to receive the positive experiences and feedback that leads to positive self-concepts. Persons with CI and impaired self concepts are apt to seek membership in groups and develop relationships with individuals that may be usurious of them, to become socially isolated, and are at increased risk of becoming depressed. This self perpetuating cycle of low self-esteem leading to negative experiences yielding even lower self-esteem needs to be altered if self-concept is to be improved.

The following case illustrates the nature of social difficulties and self concept problems for a person with CI:

Jim, a successful college football player with professional football potential, asked to be assessed at the university testing and counseling center for a suspected learning disability because he was unable to read efficiently and, therefore, was experiencing academic difficulties. During the intake interview it became apparent that he had substantial disabilities in addition to his reading disability. He, at first, reported that he was fully accepted by his full team and had many friends on the team and in the university community. However, after exploration of his social acceptance he began to explain how his team mates accommodated him and viewed him as "special" because of his differences. Further, both the coaches and other players would sometimes become annoyed with the unusual nature of his decisions because of difficulties in responding appropriately to social cues (e.g., carrying practical jokes too far) and interacting with groups (e.g., becoming easily confused in conversations or discussions and as a result responding in unusual and tangential ways). Similar difficulties were experienced in other areas of his life and contributed to the loss of his girl friend of one year, an event that distressed him greatly.

Initially, Jim did not comprehend the nature of his social difficulties, therefore, he could not develop adequate compensatory skills. The assistance he had received within the educational system focused only on his academic difficulties and led him to believe that if he could read normally the totality of his life would be normal. Limited self awareness and insight into the effects of his other difficulties impaired success in several life areas. His CI caused, not only his reading disorder, but was the cause of substantial interpersonal problems and impaired self-concept. For Jim to develop full adult capabilities, responsibilities, and group social standing, his reading *and* his personal and social difficulties were in need of treatment.

As outlined in the preceding sections, comprehensive assessment of the effects of CI, including the combined effects of multiple deficits, is critical to providing comprehensive assistance. As social workers and other professionals take a holistic approach with their clients with CI, including their social and emotional problems and strengths, they will be addressing needs their clients view as most important to their lives (Pihl & McLarnon, 1984). Increased attention to psychosocial problems and needs will frequently reveal that sexuality and sexual development are adversely affected by CI and may need preventive and remedial intervention.

COGNITIVE IMPAIRMENTS AND SEXUALITY

From childhood, sexual learning and development are influenced by psychosocial factors that, especially for persons with CI, are often contradictory and confusing. Discrepant messages require discrimination to decipher and people with CI are disadvantaged in adequately judging accurate information and acquiring correct sexual knowledge and appropriate sexual attitudes.

Sexual Knowledge, Values and Relationships

Sexual knowledge is derived from a variety of sources. As children develop, some information regarding sexuality is taught formally in contexts such as school classrooms; however, a substantial amount of sexuality learning occurs informally from the environment and in social contexts (Steptoe, 1987). Persons with CI have difficulty prioritizing and determining the relevance of information, and are disadvantaged in their ability to develop socially desirable behaviors from unstructured learning environments. For example, information taught formally in classroom settings about genital maturation may be understood, but, without specific education, a person with CI may not have the ability to discern when it is appropriate to talk about this information. This problem was demonstrated when a 12 year old girl with a moderate traumatic brain injury told her parents' friends, at a dinner party, the information she had learned about menstruation in her health class that morning.

Even in formal educational settings in which the environment is controlled, people with CI may have difficulty selectively attending to and prioritizing relevant stimuli. Even in this environment, students with CI can fail to make intended associations. This phenomenon is exemplified by the following:

As part of a social skills curriculum, Ms. Johnstone, a second grade teacher, used role playing to involve the children in simulated situations in which appropriate and inappropriate methods of problem solving were demonstrated. Though the lesson was intended to be gender neutral, Ms. Johnstone inadvertently role cast by gender, using boys to demonstrate aggressive behavior. At the conclusion of the role plays, she asked the students to explain what they had learned. When Jerry, a student with minimal brain dysfunction volunteered to share his learning with the class, he stated that it was all right for boys to talk mean, and that girls should talk nice. The other students in the class learned the intended lesson that assertiveness was preferable to aggression, but without specific feedback from the teacher, Jerry had became fixed on the gender distinctions.

This example demonstrates Jerry's need for explicit assistance to distinguish relevant from irrelevant information. Left to draw inferences on their own, people with CI are susceptible to reaching inaccurate or spurious conclusions.

Another way in which children with CI are especially susceptible to misunderstanding gender roles may occur through the use of children's literature. Several surveys of award winning picture books for children regarding sexuality and sex roles of the characters spanning the past 50 years (Dougherty & Engel, 1987; Engel, 1981; Nilsen, 1978), indicate that female characters in these books are frequently depicted in roles subservient to males, are less often than males to be depicted as main characters or to be named in book titles, and are dependent on men to be rescued, saved, or validated. These tendencies are illustrated in the award winning picture book *Mufaro's Beautiful Daughters: An African Tale* (Steptoe, 1987), in which the more subservient, subordinate and dutiful of Mufaro's two daughters married the prince and lived happily ever after while his independent, strong-willed daughter was rewarded with unhappiness. When Jenny, a young girl with CI read this, she concluded she should be passive and that marriage was the true way to gain happiness. Though all children are inundated with gender typing messages in our society, those with CI are especially susceptible to interpreting these in fixed and concrete ways that can lead to unpredictable and undesirable conclusions. Therefore, it is particularly important that people with CI receive guidance in interpreting messages.

The acquisition of personal values is an essential element in the development of sexuality. Role models can be important in developing socially appropriate values. However, determining which models best emulate values worthy of incorporation may be difficult for persons with CI and may become especially difficult when potential role models exhibit conflicting behaviors. For example, sports figures are often the objects of adoration by young people who may emulate the behaviors of their heroes. However, as in the recent case of a champion professional boxer who was convicted of rape, they may be poor examples. When this happened, Bob, an amateur boxer with MBD who idolized the fighter's rise from poverty, his fighting prowess, and his machismo became quite confused. When the fighter was arrested, Bob expressed his conviction that his hero was a victim of a sinister plot. As events progressed, he expressed such thoughts as the woman "really wanted it" or was "just after publicity." Even after the verdict was rendered, he was convinced his hero was incapable of raping anyone. Though others may have expressed similar beliefs because of distorted or sexist ideas, it was clear Bob was truly confused with the situation. Bob's social worker helped ease his confusion by contrasting socially accepted violence that occurs in boxing and contrasting it to the violence of rape in which violence is perpetrated on a victim. He was helped to articulate that people, including his hero, could have admirable qualities but also be guilty of abhorrent behavior such as rape.

For most individuals, the development of personal values is determined by strong and persistent influences during their developmental years and presumes that individuals are capable of dealing with conflicting ideas and can accommodate models of behavior that are consistent with their budding values. For a person with CI, this accommodative process may not be adequate and the individual will require guidance with interpreting and accepting models that will be consistent with and useful in their environments. The difficulties people with CI experience in gaining social acceptance and group membership, which are so important to values development (Mahoney, 1983), further complicate the development of personal values. Social impoverishment, combined with CI's cognitive deficits leaves people with CI with limited interpretive abilities and without stable peer groups, all of which can impair their values development:

Maryann, an 18 year old woman was arrested for loitering at a truck stop. When visited by a mental health social worker at the jail, it was revealed that Maryann had severe LD. Her frustrated parents reported that Maryann had spent much time in special educational classes and had been socially isolated in school. They reported that she was prone to be loud and socially inappropriate, behaviors that alienated her from peers. At about age 16, Maryann's physical development led to significant sexual attention from a group of boys in her school. She took their sexual advances as complimentary, and despite warnings from teachers and her parents, she responded with sexual enthusiasm to her new found "acceptance." Though she was eventually rejected by the group of boys, she had learned that she could gain the attention and acceptance she craved through sex. In fact, at the time of her arrest she was seeking sexual companionship from truck drivers, an activity in which she engaged frequently.

The cognitive and social consequences of Maryann's CI contributed to behaviors that were hazardous to her safety and health. Though she had been taught and could articulate healthy values, her need for social acceptance was more important to her.

Maryann's case is illustrative of the extent to which cognitive and social deficits can lead to relationship and sexual problems. A logical consequence of social non-acceptance and isolation is a tendency to seek relationships and acceptance wherever possible; even when subsequent acceptance may be injurious. The opportunities for healthy intimate relationships may be limited and the tendency to become involved in usurious relationships increased.

At the other end of the spectrum, people with CI may also alienate themselves from others. This tendency is illustrated by the case of Laura who was raised in a very religious home and who consistently angered other adolescents in her peer group by perseverating about her "righteousness" and superior "spiritual" nature, chiding them for their "worldliness." She missed few opportunities to tell her peers how to dress modestly and to avoid getting attention from boys. Her peers, both male and female, eventually refused to associate with her. Peers knew something was "wrong" but felt abused by Laura. Their reactions left Laura bereft of same-sex friendships and she had no opportunities for opposite-sex friendships.

Sexual Vulnerability and Aggression

The development of healthy sexual behavior is complicated by inconsistent and often conflicting messages from media, educational systems, role models, and peers. This is especially true given the limitations of persons with CI to reason, problem solve, and communicate effectively. The lack of consistency can contribute to actions and decisions that can cause particular difficulty for persons with CI. Two areas that may be especially problematic are sexual aggression and victimization. Behaviors may be based more on context or immediate wants than on values or rational decision making. Poor decision-making and impulsiveness put people with CI at increased risk for sexual victimization. Maryann's case is illustrative. Though she had not been forcibly sexually assaulted, she consistently placed herself in high risk environments. In addition, her case is an example of the more subtle exploitation for which people with CI are susceptible.

The increased risks of sexual victimization were demonstrated to one of the authors when providing head injury training at a prison facility. Asked to consult with prison employees assigned to a "special unit" for prisoners at high risk of victimization, the author was asked for guidance regarding one or two inmates. However, as a result of consultation, inmate records were reviewed and the prison staff reported that "virtually all the inmates" who needed protection from sexual and other victimization by separation from the regular population either had borderline mental retardation or had a history of head injuries or other CI.

Cognitive impairments can also be a contributing factor to sexual aggression. Poor impulse control, problem solving and communication deficits and difficulty in ascertaining appropriate contextual expectations can all contribute to inappropriate sexual behaviors. A mild form of this may appear as in the case of Tom who, upon reaching adolescence, began to impulsively make loud and suggestive comments in public towards women. Other, more serious implications, could include aggressive or assaultive behaviors. For example:

> John, a 28 year old married man with two children sustained a serious head injury in an automobile accident. He was comatose for 10 days and hospitalized 8 weeks. Upon returning home from the hospital, he was prone to outbursts of verbal abuse of his wife and children. In counseling, John's wife Lynn reported she felt like her husband had become more like a third child than her husband. One evening, when Lynn refused John's sexual advances, he became verbally abusive and attempted to physically force her into having sex. Lynn escaped and, as a result of the incident, John was removed from the home.

Unlike most sexual assaults, John's behavior was a result of the problems associated with his CI. After the event, he was able to develop only partial insight into the impact of his behavior. Lack of understanding or insight compounds the problem of people with CI. Victims may lack understanding of their victimization. Aggressors may also lack insights. Without assistance, people with CI are at increased risk of situations in which sexual aggression occurs, either as victims or perpetrators.

IMPLICATIONS FOR SOCIAL WORK

Social work professionals should be prepared to address the sexuality needs of their clients with CI, beginning at an early age, in a consistent manner, and with attention to the specific needs of individual clients. When multiple professionals and agencies are involved, cooperation and coordination of efforts are also important.

Interventions During Childhood and Adolescence

Sexuality education, especially when initiated in childhood is ideally proactive and preventive. Early intervention need not be distinctly sexual, but can be oriented to the development of positive self image and constructive social relationships. As children mature, education becomes increasingly sophisticated.

It is important that education and counseling interventions be developed or modified so that they meet the learning styles of CI recipients. Role plays, sociodramas, and other active participatory approaches help prepare CI clients for real life experiences. Russell and Morrill (1991) found that, for clients with CI, counseling approaches involving active client participation, such as role plays and psychodrama, were significantly more effective than traditional talk therapy in modifying behaviors and precipitating positive client actions. These participatory activities can help clients prepare to deal with real life experiences in safe learning environments and are easier for persons with CI to assimilate than textbook or other pedagogical learning activities.

Another approach to educate young people with CI includes the use of stories and picture books. Similarly, the use of drama can be helpful. Messages or themes derived from these sources can be put into contemporary social contexts and used to illustrate situations people may confront and help them develop strategies to deal with situations. As an example, the use of books that portray females as competent and capable of independence and that portray males as capable and desirous of sensitivity can be read, discussed and applied to the lives of participants. Role play and sociodrama can be used to reinforce learning. Similarly, books on sexual development and maturation can be used.

Strategy training, used to specify concrete steps people go through to complete tasks, has been demonstrated effective for assisting individuals with CI to increase functioning (Deshler, Schmaker, Lenz, & Ellis, 1984). The client is taught the steps of decision-making and task completion and how to implement the steps to complete selected objectives. This approach, for example, could be used to develop strategies to use in asking someone for a date. To prepare to do so, the person discusses such activities as what they will say, the manner in which they contact the potential date, and where they might want to go on the date. These activities help people explore options and develop plans. Strategy training is used to develop strategies for a wide range of activities, including relationship development, as well as employment management and impulse control, and can be modified to fit the developmental needs of clients.

Role playing, strategy training, drama and similar activities can all be carried out individually or in small group therapy and educational settings. Small groups are especially helpful for children and adolescents who need such explicit treatment. The social worker conducts, guides, monitors function of and processes the activities of the small group while group members benefit from the successes and mistakes of other participants.

During childhood and adolescence, most individuals with CI who receive help will do so in the special education programs of educational systems. Special education programs are designed to help students compensate for their academic problems and maximize education potentials. Special educational settings are an ideal place for social work interventions relative to the psychosocial and sexual concerns of clients with CI. Social workers have the opportunity to bolster resources and intervene in psychosocial and sexual areas through the use of activities described above. Working in conjunction with special educational teachers, they can provide valuable interventions.

The value of social work involvement in special education is enhanced because, by law, the specific needs of clients must be developed and documented in written individual education plans (IEPs). Active participation of social work professionals throughout the educational planning process, including IEP preparation, helps ensure that psychosocial and sexual needs are addressed as part of students' overall educational plans.

As social workers, classroom and special education teachers, along with students with CI and their family members work cooperatively, they will be better able to identify training needs, set goals, develop programs, and provide guidance to the students. They can also be invaluable in facilitating transitions from youth services to adult services as people with CI age into adulthood. Social workers are logical professionals to facilitate cooperation between schools, communities, and home settings and to help integrate the values and needs of families into specific client plans. Integrating family values and family members into planning increases family cooperation and contextual consistency, thereby, increasing the effectiveness of interventions.

Interventions for Adults with Cognitive Impairments

Transition services from entitlement, educational agencies to non-entitlement, adult agencies are essential in the habilitation of many clients. As a result of the Individuals with Disabilities Education Act of 1990, education agencies are now required to begin collaborating with adult services agencies beginning when the client is 16 years of age (Public Law 101-476, 1990). Transition planning provides social workers in education further opportunity to assist in the life span needs of clients as they network with multiple entities including clients, families, vocational and other social services agencies. Providers of adult services benefit from information about client strengths, needs and deficits as a result of this networking and thus, ease the difficulties of transition from child to adult services. Networking is also beneficial because it minimizes the need for clients to make cognitive shifts and helps them establish new relationships in advance of direct services, providing continuity as people transition from youth to adult services.

As people with CI reach adulthood, educational entitlement services are replaced by non-entitlement services. Emotional and behavioral concerns take precedence over educational needs. Sexuality concerns are at least as salient in adulthood as in childhood and people with CI often benefit from a range of preventive and remediative sexuality services. An example of a CI problem with sexuality implications is illustrated below:

> Sean, a 27 year old man experienced substantial academic, social, and vocational difficulties due to his CI. Despite his above average intelligence he was unable to control frustration, accurately read social cues, and prioritize routine decisions. Although he was described as kind, generous, giving and caring, he was unable to maintain sustained dating relationships. Generally, relationships were ended by women friends because of his difficulty keeping his date and time commitments. What appeared to be his lack of commitment

and thoughtlessness was actually his inability to prioritize and to make decisions, and an inability to decline requests for assistance by friends or relatives. For instance, when his father would ask for his assistance he would agree to the request even when it conflicted with dating plans. It would not occur to Sean to suggest that the task be postponed or to indicate he had a prior commitment. As a result, his relationships suffered. Through the use of strategy training, Sean was able to develop a formal structure for making decisions and to apply rehearsed responses to requests for his assistance. For example, he learned to say "I have another commitment at that time, can we do it at another time?" When he had to decide between competing events, he was taught to write down and weigh the pros and cons of each. He used this process to decide the course of action he was to take.

While this approach was relatively simple, the mental health social worker helped Sean to appropriately plan his time and prioritize decisions. He was helped to develop and maintain an intimate relationship for an extended period of time by respecting her time and feelings by monitoring his own schedule. Further, strategy training simplified and enriched his social life, family life, and vocational success through developing more positive relations with friends, family, and employers.

The above case illustrates how social interventions can have a direct impact on sexuality and intimate relationships. Other problems may be more directly sexually related as was discussed in the case of John. Some may need assistance in how to communicate within intimate relationships. Whatever the problem, the goals of treatment may be similar to clients without CI, but social workers will need to employ strategies that take into account their clients' individual needs.

CONCLUDING REMARKS

This paper has addressed the limitations in thought processes common to people with CI; limitations that can impact their ability to: control impulsiveness, reason and problem solve, gain social acceptance, maintain positive self-concepts, and communicate effectively. Although all persons with CI are unique in the specific limitations they experience, the development of sex roles, adoption of socially acceptable sexual attitudes, and the ability to establish social and intimate relationships are global concerns.

While the literature is clear that social interactions and personal relationships are seriously impacted by CI (Smith, 1991), attention to sexuality concerns has been limited. Social workers can be of vital importance in directly helping people with CI with their social and sexuality concerns, and indirectly by coordinating a continuum of services. By using the proactive and participatory interventions that have already been used effectively social workers can help people with CI develop strategies to improve their interpersonal and sexual development and functioning. Finally, social workers are critical in the development of new knowledge and interventions to enhance client sexuality.

REFERENCES

Bender, W. N. (1992). *Learning disabilities: Characteristics, identification, and teaching strategies.* Boston: Allyn and Bacon.

Bender, W. N., Bailey, D. B., Stuck, G. B., & Wyne, M. D. (1984). Relative peer status of learning disabled, educable mentally handicapped, low achieving, and normally achieving children. *Child Study Journal, 13*, 209-216.

Blalock, J. W., & Johnson, D. J. (1987). Primary concerns and group characteristics. In Johnson, D. J., & Blalock, J. W. (Eds.) *Adults with learning disabilities* (Chapter 3). Orlando: Grune & Stratton.

Carbo, M. (1983). Research in reading and learning style: Implications for exceptional children. *Exceptional Children, 49*, 486-494.

Ceci, S., Ringstorm, M., & Lea, S. (1981). Do language learning disabled children have impaired memories? In search of underlying process. *Journal of Learning Disabilities, 14*, 159-163.

Deshler, M., Schmaker, J., Lenz, B., Ellis, E. (1984). Academic and cognitive interventions of LD adolescents: Part 11. *Journal of Learning Disabilities, 17*, 170-187.

Dougherty, W. & Engel, R. (1987). An 80s look for sex equality in Caldecott winners and honor books. *The Reading Teacher, 40*, 394-398.

Engel, R. E. (1981). Is unequal treatment of females diminishing in children's picture books? *The Reading Teacher, 34*, 647-652.

Epstein, M. H., Cullinan, D., & Sternberg, L. (1977). Impulsive cognitive tempo in severe and mild learning disabled children. *Psychology in the Schools*, 14, 290-294.

Gregory, J. F., Shanahan, T., & Walberg, G. (1986). A profile of learning disabled twelfth-graders in regular classes. *Learning Disability Quarterly*, 9, 33-42.

Horn, W. F., O'Donnell, J. P., & Vitulano, L. A. (1983). Long-term follow-up studies of learning disabled persons. *Journal of Learning Disabilities*, 9, 542-554.

Kelly, J. A., Wildman, B. G., Urey, J. R., & Thurman, C. (1979). Group skills training to increase the conversational repertoire of retarded adolescents. *Child Behavior Therapy*, 1(4), 323-336.

Lezak, M., & O'Brien, K. (1990). Chronic emotional, social, and physical changes after traumatic brain injury. In, Bigler, E. (1990). *Traumatic brain injury*. Austin, TX: PRO-ED.

Mahoney, E. R. (1983). *Human sexuality*. New York: McGraw-Hill Inc.

Nilsen, A. P. (1978). Five factors contributing to the unequal treatment of females in children's picture books. *Top of the News*, 34, 255-259.

Pihl, R. O., & McLarnon, L. D. (1984). Learning disabled children as adolescents. *Journal of Learning Disabilities*, 17, 96-100.

Prigatano, G. P., & Klonoff, P. S. (1988). Psychotherapy and neuropsychological assessment after brain injury. *Journal of Head Trauma Rehabilitation*, 3(1), 45-56.

Public Law 101-467 (1990). Individuals with Disabilities Education Act.

Richey, D. D., & McKinney, J. D. (1978). Classroom behavioral style of learning disabled boys. *Journal of Learning Disabilities*, 11, 297-302.

Russell, T., & Morrill, C. (1991). Unpublished manuscript.

Smith, C. R. (1991). *Learning disabilities: The interaction of learner, task, and setting*, 2nd Ed. Boston: Allyn & Bacon.

Steptoe, J. (1987). *Mufaro's beautiful daughters: An African tale*. New York: Lathrop, Lee, and Shepard Books.

Torgesen, J. K. (1984). Memory processes in reading disabled children. *Journal of Learning Disabilities*, 18, 350-357.

Torgesen, J. K., Murphy, H., & Ivey, C. (1979). The effects of orienting task on memory performance of reading disabled children. *Journal of Learning Disability*, 12, 396-401.

Children with Special Needs: Sources of Support and Stress for Families

Deborah P. Valentine

SUMMARY. This discussion describes the sources of stress and support in the lives of twenty-five families caring for children with developmental disabilities. Utilizing the ecomap as an assessment and planning tool, four family profiles are suggested: the well-supported family; the stressed family; the isolated family; and the over-extended family. The importance of assessing the environmental stresses and social supports of parents and children with disabilities is discussed and intervention strategies are suggested.

The struggles, concerns, worries and pains experienced by parents of children with developmental disabilities do not end with the realization and acceptance that a child has a handicapping condition. Parents continue to face challenges of ongoing stresses and day to day demands of caring for a child with special needs. Regardless of the handicapping condition, parents are virtually unprepared for meeting the direct care needs of a child with developmental disabilities. It is not uncommon for parents to respond to these stresses in ways that jeopardize their own physical and emotional health and compromise the care that is given to dependent family members.

The multiple stresses that are experienced by parents who have a child with developmental disabilities and their particular vulnerability to stress are reported by parents, researchers and clinicians (Gallagher, Beckman, & Cross, 1983; Wikler, 1981; Turnbull & Turnbull, 1985). Special stress experienced by parents of children with developmental disabilities includes financial hardships resulting from their needs for special equipment, special medical care, and special programs; fatigue; multiple role demands; and critical, non-empathic attitudes and expectations of professionals. Evidence of severe stress and its consequences can be found in reports of increased suicide and divorce rates among parents of children with mental retardation (Price-Bonham & Addison, 1978). Embry (1980) and Garbarino, Brookhouser, and Authier (1987) also report disturbing evidence that children with disabilities are at greater risk for maltreatment.

Social workers have become increasingly involved in meeting the needs of children with developmental disabilities since the Equal Education for All Handicapped Children Act (Public Law 94-142) of 1975. The more recent Public Law 99-457 of 1986, an amendment of the Education of the Handicapped Act, authorizes early intervention programs for infants and toddlers with special needs from birth. The law further requires that special services involve parents and/or guardians in both the assessment and program development processes. Social workers within school systems as well as social workers within health and mental health settings, are looking for ways to facilitate parent-professional partnerships and address concerns of families with special needs consistent with the conclusion of Berger and Fowlkes (1980) that:

> Family involvement in the education of young children will work best when: (1) attention is paid to the needs of all family members, not just the young child; and (2) explicit emphasis is placed on linking the family and other social agencies and personnel in ways that utilize skills and aspirations of family network members and professionals for the future of young children. (p. 30)

The importance of assessing the social supports of families caring for children with developmental disabilities is discussed. In addition, the sources of social support and stress of 25 families caring for children with special needs are described and four family profiles are identified. Intervention strategies are also suggested.

SOCIAL SUPPORT AND STRESS

The amount of stress and the ways in which parents manage stress, influence the quality of care that both youngsters with disabilities and their siblings receive within the family. The sensitive and competent practitioner will attempt to eliminate or reduce sources of stress whenever and wherever possible.

Both clinical observations and formal research have identified an additional factor that contributes to an increased likelihood that persons can manage both acute and chronic stress: social support. Extra family resources and social supports include the "emotional, physical, informational, instrumental and material aid and assistance provided by others to maintain health and well-being, promote adaptations to life events, and foster development in an adaptive manner" (Dunst, Trivette, & Deal, 1988, p. 28).

Social isolation, for example, has been powerfully and consistently associated with increased incidence of child maltreatment (Garbarino, 1977). Support systems moderate the effects of high levels of stress on families and individuals (Cobb, 1976). Garbarino (1977) maintains that it is "the unmanageability of stress which is the most important factor and the unmanageability of the stress is a product of the mis-match between the level of stress and the availability and potency of the support systems" (p. 4).

Persons with developmental disabilities and their families depend more on enriched sources of support than others. Persons with developmental disabilities also depend on special environments for their emotional, physical and social well-being (Schilling & Schinke, 1983). Thus, the importance of identifying the spectrum of social supports available to and utilized by individuals and families with special needs is crucial to facilitate an optimal quality of life.

Two primary support system networks, informal social networks and formal support systems, can be utilized to moderate individual and family stressors. Formal support systems include both professionals and agencies that are formally organized to provide assistance to individuals and families seeking help. These include the child's school system, agencies providing services such as Easter Seals, public social service agencies, youth programs, accessible transportation systems and Special Olympics. Schilling and Schinke (1983) maintain that although the responsibility for the well-being of children with disabilities falls first on families, the extraordinary needs of persons with developmental disabilities and their families cannot be met through informal helping alone. The quality and availability of formal social supports and the degree to which they are responsive to the needs of persons with disabilities clearly impact both the individuals with special needs and their families. Formal social supports are, therefore, one factor contributing to the "habitability" of the social environment for families.

An informal social support network, on the other hand, refers to a person's relatives, friends, neighbors, co-workers, social groups and others who share material goods and services, emotional support, intimacy, affection, and information in response to both expected and non-expected life events. The importance of informal social support networks for persons with disabilities and their families cannot be overemphasized. Featherstone (1980) describes the sense of relief parents experience when they discover other parents with children with developmental disabilities. Publications such as *Exceptional Parent* and organizations such as ARC (previously Association for Retarded Citizens) and a variety of both national and local self-help organizations providing parent-to-parent support and information lend credence to the power of social connectedness. The support of family, friends and neighbors also contributes to the "habitability" of a family's social environment.

In the social worker's efforts to be most helpful to parents of children with disabilities, a critical strategy is to assess the degree of isolation and the quality of both formal and informal social supports in the environment of families. Are supports available to mediate the stress experienced by parents of children with special needs and how are these supports experienced? Are families isolated, thereby exacerbating the multiple stresses of family life? What is the quality, accessibility and availability of social supports to children with disabilities and their families? An assessment tool developed by Ann Hartman (1978) called the *ecomap* is one way to assess this.

ASSESSING CONNECTEDNESS

The ecomap is a simple paper and pencil evaluation tool developed by Ann Hartman (1978):

It maps in a dynamic way the major systems that are a part of the family's life and the nature of the family's relationships with various systems. The ecomap portrays an overview of the family in their situations; it pictures the important nurturant or conflict-laden connections between the family and the world. It demonstrates the flow of resources, or the lacks and deprivations. This mapping procedure highlights the nature of the interfaces and points to conflicts to be mediated, bridges to be built, and resources to be sought and mobilized. (Hartman, 1978, p. 377)

The ecomap also displays certain characteristics of the family. Most importantly, it describes the nature of the boundaries between family and the external world and the ease with which people and resources move across the boundary (Hartman, 1985).

The ecomap is completed by the clinician using information provided by family members. Family members are asked to identify both formal and informal social networks that exist outside the household and with whom they interact. Formal supports commonly identified by parents of children with developmental disabilities include health care systems, schools or educational systems, places of employment, and the social welfare system. Informal social supports typically identified include extended family members, neighbors, friends, and recreational and church affiliations. The clinician further asks the family to describe the quality of the relationship between family members and the social network. The connections are illustrated by drawing different kinds of lines from the social network to the family. A straight, solid line indicates a strong, supportive relationship. A straight solid line with slashes through it represents a stressful relationship. A series of dashes indicates a tenuous relationship which the family characterizes as neither supportive nor stressful. A tenuous relationship may also be one in which the quality of the relationship is characterized by the family as both supportive and stressful with neither dominating. When no line is drawn between the system and the family unit, the family has indicated that no relationship exists and the family is isolated from that particular system as a support network.

The ecomap is an especially useful tool for beginning the assessment process with parents of children with developmental disabilities. The ecomap provides families with an immediate, concise, and visual picture of where some of their difficulties lie. Parents with educational or cognitive limitations find the ecomap to be especially helpful. Frequently, parents immediately recognize by the graphic representation of the ecomap that they have become isolated and are receiving insufficient support from either formal or informal social networks. Others are struck by the number or sources of stressful connections in their lives. The use of the ecomap can be a valuable diagnostic and planning device to help social workers and families begin the problem solving process.

CAREGIVING FAMILIES

Between 1988-1991, twenty-five families were seen by the author for family assessments at a university affiliated pediatric clinic. Children are referred to the clinic for comprehensive, multidisciplinary evaluations because of concerns about developmental progress. Children receive complete medical, psychological, educational, speech and language, and auditory evaluations. In addition, the social worker on the team conducts a social history and assesses the strengths and needs of the child and his or her family. An ecomap is completed at this time and the social worker elicits a self report from parents regarding their overall feelings of isolation, stress and support.

Of the 25 families assessed in this study, 18 of the children referred were boys and seven were girls. Seventeen of the 25 children were Caucasian and eight were African Americans. The ages of the children ranged from 28 months to 17 years old. Twelve were income eligible for public health or welfare benefits and were considered to be surviving with limited financial resources. Seventeen children were evaluated and found to be functioning in the moderate to severe range of mental retardation. Four children were diagnosed as having both learning disabilities and behavioral problems. Two children were diagnosed as having severe language/communication disorders and two children had mild learning difficulties.

Although most of the children were living with both birth parents, a variety of family structures were represented in this study due to divorce, death of a parent, or adoption. Twelve of the families had three or more children. In only four families was the child evaluated an only child.

The amount and the quality of connectedness experienced by the families interviewed are reported as well as the specific sources of support and stress for families caring for children with special needs. The implications for social work practice are also discussed.

Family Connectedness

Family connectedness with systems outside the immediate household was assessed in two ways. The *number* of relationships family members maintained was calculated and the *quality* (supportive or stressful) of relationships was recorded.

Twenty-five families were interviewed. The mean number of connections between families and systems outside their families was 6.1 with a range of 3-14 relationships. Of the 25 families interviewed, nineteen of the families reported between six and nine relationships of any kind (supportive, stressful or tenuous) with either formal or informal support systems outside their immediate households. Three of the 25 families reported five or fewer connections with systems outside their immediate households and three families reported ten or more connections with others outside their households.

Based on the distribution and the clinical evaluations of the family assessment interviews, four tentative family profiles are identified by the author: the *well supported family*; the *stressed family*; the *isolated family*; and the *overextended family*. It is important to emphasize that the following descriptions are based on clinical impressions and provide merely a suggested descriptive clustering for the assessment of families caring for children with developmental disabilities. The descriptions are intended only as a beginning point from which to conduct further qualitative and quantitative research into the social support networks of families.

Well supported families. Of the 19 families that reported between 6-9 connections outside their immediate households, 14 indicated that they had more supportive relationships than stressful ones. This represents more than half of the entire sample and is identified by the author as the well supported family. These families tended to report that they received the help and encouragement they needed most of the time. During the interviews, these families communicated a general sense of optimism and contentment and reported feeling a sense of belonging. Although all of the families in this group also reported stressful relationships with one or more systems outside their households, the overall, general life outlook reported was positive and they felt that stress was manageable.

Frequently, social work services are not recommended for families who are well supported unless they are directly requested by the family or problem areas are identified within the family or with a particular environmental system. Often, well supported families make excellent resources for other families who are struggling with the care of children with developmental disabilities. Members of well supported families are ideal natural helpers.

Stressed families. Five of the families reporting between 6-9 connections outside their immediate households (20% of the entire sample) experienced more stressful relationships with others than they did supportive relationships. These stressed families indicated during the interviews that they experienced frequent symptoms of stress such as chronic fatigue, ill health or physical complaints such as headaches and back aches, sleep problems and/or irritability. During the interviews, family members indicated that they frequently felt anxious or confused. Despite the existence of supportive relationships, the intensity and the number of stressful relationships between members of the household and outside systems were so great that supportive relationships did not sufficiently buffer these families from stress. Every family who reported a predominance of stressful relationships in their environments also reported that they frequently felt angry and hostile.

Families reporting more stressful than supportive affiliations and families reporting intensely stressful affiliations may respond eagerly to the social worker's offer to mediate conflict or assume an advocacy role when appropriate. Reducing the number and kinds of stressful relationships and replacing them with supportive ones are additional intervention strategies for the stressed family. In some families, stress reduction classes or relaxation exercises may be suggested.

Isolated families. The three families reporting five or fewer connections with systems outside their immediate households are characterized as isolated families. A concern shared by parents caring for children with special needs is the tendency to withdraw from social interactions because they feel "different," "tired," "overwhelmed," or because they feel rejected by others. Families that reported few connections of either a supportive or stressful nature expressed feelings of helplessness, sadness and loneliness. These families frequently felt helpless in the face of stress and several parents reported occasional incidents of extreme tension and even rage.

For the family characterized by isolation, referrals to parent support groups, sibling support groups, education classes or other *appropriate and relevant* informal and formal support systems are indicated. It is crucial that the social work practitioner carefully assess the specific individualized needs of family members before making recommendations and referrals. Because of the amount of time, energy, and emotional risk involved, careful selection of supports for isolated families is very important.

Overextended families. The fourth identified profile is the overextended family. Three families reported 10 or more connections with systems outside their immediate household. In each of these three families, more supportive relationships were reported than stressful relationships, however, the families differed from the well supported families in some important ways. First, these families identified so many responsibilities and interactions with others outside their families that time and energy became a scarce resource. During family assessment interviews, family members reported feeling overwhelmed and tired (not unlike the stressed families). Feelings of frustration and moodiness were also frequently reported. Parents indicated that they just did not have enough time to do everything that needed to get done. Like the stressed families, the overextended families reported physical complaints; however, these physical complaints were typically not chronic. Instead, acute periods of illnesses were reported that literally "shut down" any outside activities for periods of days or even weeks. Members of overextended families also did not describe themselves as angry; rather, they were more likely to characterize themselves as frantic or suffering from occasional feelings of inadequacy.

A social worker may offer help to the family that is overextended by assisting family members in identifying the necessity and importance of each relationship. The practitioner, for example, may act as an advocate on behalf of the family to other professionals who are placing additional or unreasonable demands on family members for their time (e.g., additional tutoring, speech or physical therapy, or recreational activities). For the family who is already overextended, a referral to a parent support group, for example, is inappropriate. The social worker may also encourage families who have overextended themselves to prioritize their activities and reduce the number of commitments they have.

In addition to the quantity and quality of connections which families caring for children with special needs report on the ecomap, the specific types of connections are also identified and provide useful information for the social work practitioner.

Specific Sources of Support and Stress

The ecomap revealed important sources of support and stress as identified by the 25 families interviewed. Twenty-one different systems were reported. The most frequently mentioned are listed in Table 1.

Parents reported that support from their places of employment was extremely important since the special needs of their children frequently meant that they must miss work to attend to the special needs of their children (evaluations, appointments and/or ill health). When the support was unavailable, parents reported a constant tension between their roles as workers and their roles as parents.

The extended maternal family was considered to be an important source of support for most families. Fifteen families indicated that the maternal family was a source of support whereas seven families indicated that the maternal family was a source of stress. Nine families, on the other hand, indicated that paternal family members were a source of support and six families indicated a stressful relationship. Although not recorded on the Table, all four divorced parents indicated that their ex-spouses were a source of stress. Parents who did not have support of extended family reported that they felt misunderstood by family members and indicated that they be-

TABLE 1
SOURCES OF SUPPORT AND STRESS FOR FAMILIES

	SUPPORT	TENUOUS	STRESS	TOTAL # OF FAMILIES
MOTHER'S WORK	6	2	2	10
FATHER'S WORK	12	2	3	17
MATERNAL FAMILY	15	2	7	24
PATERNAL FAMILY	9	3	7	19
FRIENDS	6	1	1	8
NEIGHBORS	1	0	4	5
CHURCH	9	2	1	12
SCHOOL	9	1	9	19
HEALTH CARE	7	2	4	13
OTHER PROVIDERS	9	4	2	15
HOUSING	1	1	5	7
TRANSPORTATION	3	0	2	5

TOTAL NUMBER OF FAMILIES = 25

lieved their parenting abilities were being judged and criticized. The parents who did receive support from family members, on the other hand, reported receiving help from extended family in child care, transportation, financial support and emotional support.

Church affiliation was also very important for most of the families interviewed. Nine families indicated that their churches were very supportive. Their children with disabilities were welcomed by the congregations and allowed to participate in youth activities. Parents who found their church affiliations to be supportive also indicated that church members were accepting and non-judgmental and offered both practical and emotional support. Four of the families, however, stated that they no longer attended church because the responsibilities to their children with special needs made church participation difficult or inconvenient (e.g., no child care or transportation). One family indicated that their church affiliation was stressful because their church was unwilling to allow their child to participate in its youth activities and had a general attitude of "rejection" of the child.

It is interesting to note that when families mentioned neighbors, four of the five families reported that they were a source of stress. That is, most families did not consider their neighbors an important enough affiliation to mention; when they did, they tended to be reported as stressful. Parents reported that neighborhood children teased their children; their families were ostracized from neighborhood activities; or their neighbors were criminally involved or perceived as dangerous. Evaluating neighborhoods and working with families to improve relationships when possible and develop positive relationships where none exist can be an important source of help for many families caring for children with developmental disabilities.

The interaction between school and family was extraordinarily important for all families who had children attending school. The home-school relationship is one of the most widely recognized interfaces between the family and the community. Garbarino (1982) maintains that "the congruence between home and school can have a large and significant effect upon child development . . . A strong home-school mesosystem is a set of multiple and mutually respectful relationships between families and school officials," a conclusion supported by the data (p. 160). Parents who indicated that their children were receiving adequate educational services in a nurturing environment reported much less overall stress than families who expressed dissatisfaction with their children's educational programs. Parents who indicated that the schools attended by their children did not provide what they considered adequate, respectful, or sufficient educational services reported extraordinary stress. These parents were frequently involved in multiple activities geared towards pressuring schools to provide them with complete information and provide appropriate services. Parents reporting stressful relationships with schools indicated that they felt that schools were "not interested in my child," and had a "hostile and blaming attitude towards us." These parents also felt that they had no advocate in the schools and reported feeling alone and isolated in their quests to meet their children's needs.

Health care services were of significant concern to most families caring for children with developmental disabilities. Families reporting stressful relationships with health care providers were concerned about attitudes and lack of knowledge of physicians and nurses about children with handicapping conditions. The financial cost of health care was also identified as being a significant stress. Other families indicated that their health care providers were a very supportive part of their lives—depending on them not only for health care but for emotional support and help with decision-making as well.

A wide range of other service providers were listed as supportive to parents. These included both private and public agencies such as Easter Seals; Department of Mental Retardation; ARC; Social Security Administration; advocacy groups; adoption agencies; and parent support groups. For the most part, these service providers were considered to be helpful to the families by providing needed financial assistance, equipment for their children, and/or emotional support.

Five families indicated that housing was a primary source of stress in their families' lives. Housing which was too small or did not have specialized construction such as ramps or doorways to accommodate the children's special equipment was considered stressful. Other families indicated that they did not have plumbing or lived in unsafe neighborhoods.

Two families mentioned transportation as a major source of stress. Neither family had a car nor was public transportation available to them. Parents indicated that this isolated them from potential sources of support such as religious services, school conferences and meetings, health care appointments and friends.

DISCUSSION

Stressful connections with one's social environment can be due to a variety of factors. Physical barriers and practical restraints, fragmentation of the social service delivery system or the unavailability of quality programs may prevent individuals with developmental disabilities and their families from building and making full use of social networks (Schilling & Schinke, 1983). Ironically, some persons most in need of social supports may also behave in ways that inhibit positive affiliations. Family members caring for children with developmental disabilities expressed being too tired, busy, or emotionally overwhelmed to seek out or maintain services or relationships. The number and intensity of demands on any family can be enormous. It is not surprising that without the efforts of family members and the community, isolation or conflict might result.

The social worker can play an important role in the lives of families with special needs. An outreach effort that emphasizes family strengths and empowerment can contribute to the building of positive relationships between social services, the community and the family. Furthermore, the social worker is in an excellent position to facilitate the development of additional supportive relationships with and on behalf of families.

One strategy may include the improvement of the quality of existing relationships between family members and both formal and informal social networks. Empowering families to change stressful connections to supportive connections by talking and explaining situations to immediate neighbors, for example, may benefit families. Work directed towards developing and promoting the accessibility of supportive social networks (parent support groups, neighborhood organizations, respite care) is another important strategy for intervening with families and advocating on their behalf.

Families and professionals can also work together and use the ecomap to evaluate progress over time. An increase in supportive relationships and a decrease in relationships characterized as stressful, for example, would be an indication of positive change. In another family, a reduction of relationships and activities would be considered progress.

The sources of support and stress identified by the 25 families in this study were quite diverse. Families reported utilizing a wide variety of formal and informal social networks for support and assistance. The amount and sources of stress as well as the amount and sources of supportive relationships are important factors in the overall care of children with developmental disabilities. The social worker using a comprehensive, ecological approach will strengthen social supports in families' environments while attempting to reduce the effect of stressors and isolation. Utilization of the ecomap as a planning, assessment and evaluation tool with families caring for children with developmental disabilities can contribute to this effort.

REFERENCES

Berger, M. & Fowlkes, M.A. (1980). Family intervention project: A family network model for serving young handicapped children. *Young Children, 34*(4), 22-32.

Cobb, S. (1976). Social support as a moderator of life stress. *Psychosomatic Medicine, 38*, 300-314.

Dunst, C., Trivette, C., & Deal, A. (1988). *Enabling and empowering families.* Cambridge, MA: Brookline Books.

Embry, L. (1980). Family support for handicapped pre-school children at risk for abuse. In J. Gallagher (Ed.), *New directions for exceptional children*, San Francisco.

Featherstone, H. (1980). *A difference in the family.* N.Y.: Basic Books, Inc.

Gallagher, J.J., Beckman, P., & Cross, A.H. (1983). Families of handicapped children: Sources of stress and its amelioration. *Exceptional Children, 50*(1), 10-19.

Garbarino, J. (1977). The human ecology of child maltreatment: A conceptual model for research. *Journal of Marriage and the Family, 39*, 721-736.

Garbarino, J. (1982). *Children and families in the social environment.* NY: Aldine de Gruyter.

Garbarino, J., Brookhauser, P.E., & Authier, K. (1987). *Special children/Special risks: The maltreatment of children with disabilities,* NY: Aldine de Gruyter.

Hartman, A. (1978). Diagrammatic assessment of family relationships. *Social Casework, 59*(8), 465-76.

Hartman, A. (1985). Practice in adoption. In J. Laird and A. Hartman (Eds.), *A handbook of child welfare* (pp. 667-692). NY: The Free Press.

Price-Bonham, S. & Addison, R. (1978). Families and mentally retarded children: Emphasis on the father. *The Family Coordinator, 27*, 221-230.

Schilling, R.F. & Schinke, S.P. (1983). Social support networks in developmental disabilities. In J.K. Whittaker & J. Garbarino (Eds.), *Social support networks: Informal helping in the human services* (pp. 383-404). NY: Aldine Publishing.

Turnbull, H.R. & Turnbull, A. (1985). *Parents speak out: Then and now,* London: Charles E. Merrill.

Wikler, L. (1981). Chronic stresses of families of mentally retarded children. *Family Relations, 30*, 281-288.

The Parent with Mental Retardation:
Rights, Responsibilities and Issues

Barbara Y. Whitman
Pasquale J. Accardo

SUMMARY. Adults with mental retardation living in the community are marrying and having children. Many are experiencing significant problems in their role as parents. Legal, professional and programmatic supports for some adults lag behind need. This article reviews legal and ethical issues surrounding this growing population. The experience of a model pilot parenting program is presented. Finally, recommendations for future efforts in this area are presented.

The issue of sexuality and persons with mental retardation is inextricably linked to the issues of marriage, childbearing, and, ultimately, parenting. Mental retardation of the mother is a recognized risk factor for neglect of the medical, emotional and cognitive needs of her children (Shaw & Wright, 1960; Madsen, 1979; Schilling, Schinke, Blythe, & Barth, 1982; Gillberg & Geijer-Karlsson, 1983). Studies regarding the quality of parenting of fathers with mental retardation are sparse. The questions of whether persons with mental retardation should be allowed to marry, have children, and whether they should be allowed to parent have been debated for centuries (Hill, 1950; Bass, 1963). The debate continues; however, normalization and deinstitutionalization of persons with mental retardation are facts. Whether or not they "should" do so, persons with mental retardation are in fact marrying, having children, and parenting (Whitman, Graves, & Accardo, 1987). The number of parents with mental retardation is increasing among the professional caseloads of pediatricians, social workers, juvenile court authorities and school personnel.

123

The answer to the question, "Can persons with mental retardation learn to be good parents?" is neither simple nor obvious. The capacity to nurture is not dependent on intelligence, for if intelligence alone predicted the ability to nurture, there would be no parents of normal intelligence guilty of child abuse or neglect. Yet the desire to have and raise a child may not be enough if a parent cannot adequately care for a child due to an inability to provide routine feedings, to read a thermometer, or administer medications correctly because they are unable to read or to tell time; or have cognitive limitations that may make the use of transportation to medical or other service facilities impossible. By virtue of their own limitations, parents with mental retardation sometimes engage in benign neglect of their children. This paper will briefly review some of the legal, service, and ethical issues regarding the parent with mental retardation.

THE RIGHT TO MARRY

Marriage is an inalienable legal right for most Americans, however, for persons with mental retardation, statutes prohibiting marriage have been the norm. As recently as 1977, 38 states and the District of Columbia prohibited or seriously limited the right of persons with mental retardation to marry; most of these laws had been enacted within the previous decade, and most still stand (Marafino, 1990a). The intent behind these statutes is threefold: (1) to protect persons who have mental retardation, (2) to prevent procreation by persons who have mental retardation, and (3) to protect those without disabilities from marriage to a spouse with mental retardation.

The rationale for protecting persons with mental retardation requires further explanation. Marriage is a legally constituted contract and assumes competency. If an individual who enters into a contract is deemed to be "incompetent" the contract becomes void. A marriage declared void impacts on the property rights of the participants and may raise questions about the "legitimacy" of any children born to the union. Doubt about parentage can lead to denial of rightful supports, inheritances, entitlements and other such benefits that accrue to "legitimate" offspring. The intent of these laws is to prevent the harm that accrues from having a marriage declared a void contract.

The second rationale for prohibiting individuals with mental retardation from marrying is not so benign. The prohibition of marriage of persons with mental retardation is one strategy for preventing them from having children who will become social and economic burdens to the state. While initially formulated on the basis of inaccurate and unsubstantiated eugenics theories, some laws subject adults with mental retardation with penalties for procreating, penalties that may include losing custody of their children. The basis of the eugenics argument is the assumption that "mental defectives beget mental defectives." Such arguments suggest that all (or most) mental retardation is genetic or familial and that preventing procreation by those with retardation will eliminate or at least significantly decrease mental retardation in future generations. To the contrary, mental retardation is heterogeneous in etiology, including genetic as well as non-genetic causes (Accardo & Capute, 1991). Among people whose mental retardation is genetic in origin, reproduction is less likely, for the damage of the genetic insult often impacts the reproductive as well as cognitive system. Thus the eugenics argument is seriously flawed. For those parental cases of mental retardation that are nongenetic in origin, eugenics arguments fly in the face of data. For example, one recent study examined 107 children from 79 families in which one or both parents was identified with mental retardation. Of the 107 children, approximately a third (31%) were themselves diagnosed as having mental retardation. Another third exhibited some developmental delays, but most of their delays were remediated with intervention. This was particularly true in those age six and over and is thus interpretable as secondary to the child's home environment. The remaining third exhibited no cognitive deficits (Accardo & Whitman, 1990). Thus while this sample of children had a significantly higher proportion of mental retardation than would be expected in general population, the numbers in no way support an unrestricted form of the eugenics argument. More recently, the issue of sterilization has received renewed attention (Committee on Bioethics, 1990; ACOG Committee, 1990). While the basis of current sterilization arguments is less toxic than those of the eugenics era, the thrust remains the same–persons with mental retardation should not be having children and therefore should be surgically sterilized.

The third reason given for limiting persons with mental retardation from marrying is based on the assumption that those with mental retardation are unfit to be spouses. One need only look at current divorce statistics to perceive discrimination in this argument. With nearly one-half of U.S. marriages ending in divorce, the supply of mismatched spouses certainly exceeds the number of persons with mental retardation. Nonetheless, laws such as these remain on the books in most jurisdictions today. However, for many adults with mental retardation, the right to marry is an issue legally, psychologically and physiologically different from the right to bear children and parent. The number of never married single parents continues to increase both in the population at large and in adults with mental retardation.

PARENTAL RIGHTS OF PERSONS WITH MENTAL RETARDATION

The laws and policies concerning parental rights for persons with mental retardation have evolved as the courts have acknowledged that rights afforded other parents have been denied to persons with mental retardation. Rulings have supported that mental retardation per se is not a valid reason for denying parental rights. A brief review of relevant legal rulings follows.

By culture, history, tradition and law, parents' rights to the custody and control of their offspring have been considered sacrosanct. Constitutional support of these rights and to family integrity are recognized by a series of Supreme Court decisions under the due process clause of the Fourteenth Amendment. Despite this support, federal, state and case law have had to deal with the issues of inadequate and inappropriate parenting as well as with the often conflicting rights involved ensuring children's safety and best interests and supporting parents' rights and family integrity. Until the early 1970s, parental rights weighed more heavily than children's interests–to the extent that children were considered similar to property that could be contested in divorce proceedings. The enactment of statutes for temporary and permanent termination of parental rights coupled with laws enabling states to intervene to protect the health, safety and well-being of its children from abusive and neglectful parents heralded a legal shift toward weighting the best interests of children separately from parental rights.

While providing statutory pathways for temporary and permanent cessation of parental rights, the law recognizes abuse and neglect based on parental mental disability as differently than that found in parents without disabilities. Nonetheless, while acknowledging that there is generally no intent to harm, parents with mental retardation who are guilty of child maltreatment often are treated more harshly by court systems. They are treated as incapable of rehabilitation and their children are more likely to be permanently removed with no effort to provide support or treatment (Retarded Parents in Legal Proceedings, 1979). Too often parents with mental retardation have been treated as mentally ill rather than cognitively limited. Little attention or understanding is given to actual levels of competence, ability, or desires to parent. Based on laws governing forced (no parental consent) adoption, parents who are mentally retarded have had children removed from their care (often immediately after birth) and placed for adoption solely on the basis of parental mental retardation. The severity of mental retardation, the capacity to parent, the ability to give informed consent, and the existence of extended family supports are not often considered (Brakel, Parry, & Weiner, 1985).

The trends toward deinstitutionalization and mainstreaming throughout the 1970s and 1980s, coupled with the more recent goal of total community living, contribute to increasing numbers of adults with mental retardation that reside in communities and have children (Whitman, Graves, & Accardo, 1987). Thus, in the past decade, the courts have adjudicated an increasing number of child protective cases in which one or both parents have mental retardation. This has forced a review of the statutory support for denying custodial and parental rights to parents with mental retardation. It is now firmly established that mental retardation alone is not sufficient legal justification for a permanent termination of parental rights (Marafino, 1990b). A case must be made that mental retardation sufficiently impairs parental functioning such that to remain in the parent's care causes or holds potential harm to the child, and that the basis for that impairment is irremediable with available intervention.

That persons with mental retardation are capable of parenting given the right circumstances and adequate supports is becoming well documented in the literature (Tymchuk & Andron, 1990; Whitman, Graves & Accardo, 1990). That these parents are under significant stress and have serious problems with parenting is also well documented (Schilling et al., 1982; Accardo & Whitman 1990; Seagull & Scheurer, 1986). In addition, many parents with mental retardation face such additional problems as a poverty level income, lack of vocational skills or job training, inadequate parenting models, isolation from extended families, lack of knowledge about public resources, and in many cases, a limited range of experiences (Whitman & Accardo, 1990). Thus, for many adults with mental retardation, the ability to provide adequate parenting over time depends on the presence of long term support and involvement with programs and agencies designed to facilitate adequate parenting. Specifically, parents with mental retardation may need long-term support in those areas of child-rearing that require complex cognitive input and abilities. Unfortunately, few resources are available to help adults with mental retardation deal with such problems (Crain & Millor, 1978).

PROGRAMMATIC RESPONSES

From the middle to late 1980s, several pilot programs attempted to address the needs of parents with mental retardation (Whitman, Graves & Accardo, 1990; Tymchuk & Andron, 1990; Gil & McKenna, undated). The following discussion focuses on the authors' experiences with an intervention program designed to support and enhance the parenting skills of families headed by one or more parents with mental retardation.

Parents Learning Together (PLT) involved 4 days a week of interactive, center-based instruction for both parents and their children over a period of one to several years. Criteria for entry into the program included a documented parental intelligence quotient (IQ) of 69 or less, residence in the city of St. Louis, and either a pregnancy or a preschool child in the home. The program was free to participants. Referral sources included both the Mental Retardation-Developmental Disability and the Child Welfare service networks. Twenty-three families (comprised of 23 mothers with mental retardation, three fathers with mental retardation, and 65 children) were enrolled during the first two years of the program (1983-1984). Maternal ages ranged from 17 to 41 years; IQs ranged from 35 to 69 with a mean of 50.6. A number of competency based pre-test and post-test measures were utilized.

A center-based program model was employed so that parents with mental retardation could have opportunities to meet other parents. Goals of the program included (1) opportunities for socialization experiences for parents; (2) parental participation in a self-help/ support group and social network of parents; and (3) opportunities for socialization experiences for their children. Trained volunteers were used to supervise the children in the center during the parents' classes. The children were also available for the interactive portions of PLT that focused on parenting skills. Moreover, the volunteers served as role models for both the parents and the children. The center-based programming was supplemented by follow-up home visits of one hour duration twice each week. The follow-up visits were designed to facilitate transfer of learning from the center to the home setting.

Teaching methods of the *Parents Learning Together* program included modeling, role-playing, observing, practicing, discussing, and repetition. In all parent training, a plan-do-recall strategy modified from the cognitively oriented curriculum originally developed for children (Weikert, Hohmann, & Banet, 1979) was employed. Teachers verbally articulated the task to be accomplished (plan) and the sequence of activities necessary to complete the task (do). Students then completed the tasks with the teacher and the teacher reviewed the steps of the activity with the parents' participation (recall). Sequences were continually repeated in this fashion. In each succeeding repetition, the parents gradually took over more responsibility for the sequences until they were capable of independent task completion. This strategy was necessary both for learning

130 SEXUALITY AND DISABILITIES

and for providing precise guidelines for parents with mental retardation who were encouraged to use these same strategies with their children.

Training content was developed in a self-contained, modular format. Learning in each module was assessed using a pre-test post-test format. The modules covered such areas as child development and child care, personal and child hygiene, medical care, time concepts, children's basic needs, parent-child interaction, parent-made toys, child safety, planning and organizing a daily routine and good nutrition (Graves, Graves, Haynes, Rice, & Whitman, 1990). Time for parents to meet together as a group was included to cover such activities as discussion, learning, socialization, modeling of parenting skills by staff, and observation of client interaction with one or more of their children. In addition, an individualized learning contract was developed for each participating parent and one-on-one supervision routinely provided.

A number of problems emerged. By definition, parents with mental retardation are persons who have reached adulthood with a condition that has limited both their ability to develop skills and their range of achieved adaptive behaviors. Because of their ages, many parent participants did not benefit in any substantial way from the educational mandates of P.L. 94-142, the Education for All Handicapped Children Act passed in 1975. This law mandated free public education for all handicapped children. Prior to that time, special education services were sporadically available and inconsistent in goals and quality. Thus, the curriculum and programming of PLT anticipated a number of difficulties commonly experienced by parents with mental retardation. These included issues related to poverty, lack of adequate housing, lack of basic social, communication, daily living and vocational skills, lack of adequate medical and health care, lack of transportation, family conflict and inadequate parenting skills. In addition, some of the specific cognitive problems that were encountered included: language problems, problems with organizing and sequencing, overgeneralization and undergeneralization, low self-esteem, an inordinate desire to please, inability to read social cues, inability to use nonverbal cues appropriately, sporadic attendance, and other specific learning disabilities that further limited skills. Many untreated medical and dental problems were also discovered by program staff. One mother, for example, was discovered to have a previously undiagnosed 80% hearing loss. Social problems detected by the staff included previously unidentified spouse abuse that was perceived as expected in relationships by some participants. Many of the parents had been receiving no social services prior to the PLT program. Some had been served through the educational or sheltered workshop systems prior to the birth of their children, but once pregnant or married, they were deemed ineligible for such services. Having been excluded from the Mental Retardation-Developmental Disability service network and being uninformed regarding the child welfare service network, many program participants were without service support. Often basic information regarding help and service availability was missing from the parents' fund of information. Specific problems noted included a lack of knowledge of available services; lack of knowledge regarding service application processes and procedures; and lack of knowledge about costs of services. Additional problems noted were an inability to fill out service need applications due to an inability to read; an inability to tell time or read calendar dates so that appointments to apply for services were missed; an inability to use a telephone or public transportation; and reluctance to seek help due to embarrassment regarding what others might think about their limitations. While some of the parents were unable to recognize a need for help, others had unsuccessfully sought help in the past and refused to seek further help due to a perceived insensitivity of service personnel to their special needs. A final dynamic occurred on more than one occasion. Often PLT parent participants needed help on a crisis basis when many service agencies were not open. By the time usual service hours arrived, the situation had escalated to extreme proportions and other agencies became involved (such as the local police) in taking remediative, and sometimes punitive, rather than preventive actions.

Once trust was established with human service workers at agencies, participating parents frequently overtaxed existing social support systems. In part, this tendency reflected the psychological and social crises routinely and continually experienced by parents with mental retardation. Several times, program staff had to find apartments and help move families on short notice. In one case, toxic lead levels had been discovered in the family's home. In another situation, power and water had been disconnected–an event that could have led to illness and possible removal of their children. Other examples of staff intervention included acquiring food; helping a parent locate a missing Social Security Insurance check; and intervening with an unscrupulous salesperson who was victimizing one of the parents. During the first year of the program, ten of the participating families were rendered temporarily homeless. Although it is not appropriate to generalize from PLT participating families to the general population of parents with mental retardation, the fact that almost one-half of the PLT families experienced homelessness during the first year is very troubling. The PLT experience supports the belief that homeless persons and families with mental retardation are an unidentified and underserved group (Whitman, Accardo, Boyert, & Kendagor, 1990).

Despite multiple problems and crises, many of the parents significantly improved their parenting skills and adult-child interactions and were able to establish networks of friends and professionals on whom they could rely. Many of these adults were able to break a cycle of abuse that had begun when they themselves were abused as children. Prior to the training and due to their own cognitive limitations, they were often unable to identify abuse. For most participating adults, it was assumed by their caregivers that parenting would not be a relevant issue. Preparation for parenting was virtually non-existent. When faced with the parenting role, there was little on which participants could rely. If they experienced abuse in their childhoods, the cycle of abuse was often perpetuated. The program was instrumental in interrupting this cycle by offering more appropriate alternatives.

RECOMMENDATIONS

While much attention has been focused recently on the legal rights of persons with mental retardation to marry and have appropriate sexual relationships, the rights to bear and parent children have been considered secondary to the rightful opportunity for these individuals to express love, give caring and affection, build a partnership, and satisfy sexual needs. There has been little attention given to resolving the conflicting needs and rights of adults with mental retardation to be sexually active and bear children with the needs and rights of their children. Brodeur (1990) concluded that:

> Developing an appropriate social environment for individuals with mental retardation means creating an environment where the least restraints are present. Environments of least restraint do not maximize freedom in an unbridled sense, but are designed to help individuals achieve their fullest possible potential. . . . Many persons with mental retardation are able to express love and affection and to pursue healthy interdependent relationships. The right to marriage, however, does not necessarily include a right to parenting. When it comes to children in the family setting of a couple with mental retardation, the rights or needs of the children will have to be carefully balanced against the rights and needs of the parents. (p. 194)

To guide decision making in this area, Brodeur (1990) proposes a framework of ethical principles to be employed to help decision-makers think through the issues involved in fostering or terminating parental rights. These include the following: (1) family units are to be upheld, promoted and developed; (2) children are not chattel and their rights need to be developed and respected; (3) children's problems are not confined to those of children of parents with mental retardation; (4) difficulties with parenting must be faced and may require societal intervention; (5) criteria for successful parenting need to be developed and not assumed; (6) children sometime need others to make difficult decisions for them; (7) children's long term needs cannot be sacrificed for short term adult gains; (8) one must distinguish the marital rights of persons with mental retardation from the parental rights of persons with mental retardation.

The translation of these principles into working guidelines has yet to be fully accomplished. In acting to ensure that adults who are mentally retarded have the same guarantees of freedom as any other citizen, we place ourselves in an ethical bind when we must then rule that the best interests of the child require removal from those same adults solely because of lesser intellectual ability to meet and cope with life's demands.

Adults with mental retardation living in the community are having children and many are experiencing significant problems fulfilling their roles as parents. They have the legally sanctioned right to have children. But legally sanctioned rights do not translate into the capacity for responsible action. Thus it is left to those who work with adults with mental retardation and to the community at large to develop the programmatic supports to enable them to enjoy their rights while continuing to be responsible for meeting the needs and rights of the children involved. Programming adjusted to address parenting needs identified in mothers and fathers with mental retardation is not readily available. Yet scarcity of resources is not a valid reason to occasion family breakup that may not be in the best interests of the child or the adult. A number of supportive services currently available for most parents can be expanded to meet the needs of parents with special needs. These include: respite services for parents, day care for children, parent to parent networking and support, adult day services, transportation to and from services, sheltered workshop with day care and parenting services, recreation and leisure services for special needs families, family life education, counseling, money management, supervised and supported family housing and homemaker services.

Mental retardation is neither a necessary nor a sufficient reason to exclude individuals from parenting. The question with regard to the parenting problems of persons with mental retardation would seem to be not whether they should parent, but under what conditions they shouldn't parent. And with this question we come full circle to the thesis that the capacity to parent is not predictable by IQ alone. Thus we are left with the same questions raised previously by Brodeur (1990):

> One can question whether parents with mental retardation are being held to a different standard than other parents and the answer may be yes; perhaps the question should be asked whether other parents should be held to the same standard that parents with mental retardation are expected to meet. (p. 202)

Further research on the impact on both parent and child of various situational parameters other than the degree of parental mental retardation is needed.

REFERENCES

Accardo, P.J. & Capute, A.J. (1991). Mental Retardation. In A.J. Capute & P.J. Accardo (Eds.), *Developmental disabilities in infancy and childhood* (pp. 431-639). Baltimore: Paul H. Brookes Publishing Co.

Accardo, P.J., Whitman, B.Y. (1990). Children of parents with mental retardation: Problems and diagnoses. In B.Y. Whitman & P.J. Accardo (Eds). *When a parent is mentally retarded* (pp. 123-131). Baltimore: Paul H. Brookes Publishing Co.

ACOG Committee American Academy of Pediatrics. (1990). Sterilization of women who are mentally handicapped. *Pediatrics, 85* (5), 869-871.

Bass, M.S. (1963). Marriage, parenthood and prevention of pregnancy. *American Journal of Mental Deficiency, 68* (3), 318-333.

Brakel, S., Parry, F., & Weiner, B. (1985). *The mentally disabled and the law* (3rd ed.). Chicago: American Bar Foundation.

Brodeur, D. (1990). Parents with mental retardation and developmental disabilities: Ethical issues in parenting. In B.Y. Whitman & P.J. Accardo (Eds.), *When a parent is mentally retarded* (pp. 191-202). Baltimore: Paul H. Brookes Publishing Co.

Committee on Bioethics American Academy of Pediatrics. (1990). Sterilization of women who are mentally handicapped. *Pediatrics, 85* (5), 868.

Crain, L.S. & Millor, G.K. (1978). Forgotten children: Maltreated children of mentally retarded parents. *Pediatrics, 61,* 130-132.

Gil, L. & McKenna, D. (Undated). *Parenting skills curriculum: A curriculum for mentally handicapped parents of young children.* Seattle, WA: Northwest Center Infant Development Program.

Gillberg, C. & Geijer-Karlsson, M. (1983). Children born to mentally retarded women: A 1-21 Year Follow-Up Study of 41 Cases. *Psychological Medicine, 13,* 891-894.

Graves, B., Graves, D., Haynes, Y., Rice, G., & Whitman, B. (1990). Parents learning together II: Selected modules from the curriculum. In B.Y. Whitman & P.J. Accardo (Eds.), *When a parent is mentally retarded.* Baltimore: Paul H. Brookes Publishing.

Hill, I.B. (1950). Sterilizations in Oregon. *American Journal of Mental Deficiency, 54,* 399-403.

Madsen, M. K. (1979). Parenting classes for the mentally retarded. *Mental Retardation, 17,* 195-196.

Marafino, K. (1990a). The right to marry for persons with mental retardation. In B.Y. Whitman & P.J. Accardo (Eds.), *When a parent is mentally retarded.* Baltimore: Paul H. Brookes Publishing Co. (pp. 149-161).

Marafino, K. (1990b). Parental rights of persons with mental retardation. In B.Y. Whitman & P.J. Accardo (Eds.), *When a parent is mentally retarded* (pp. 163–189). Baltimore: Paul H. Brookes Publishing Co.

Michelson, P. (1947). The feebleminded parent: A study of 90 family cases. *American Journal of Mental Deficiency, 51,* 644-653.

Retarded parent in neglect proceedings. (1979). The erroneous assumption of parental inadequacy. *Stanford Law Review, 31,* 385-401.

Schilling, R.F., Schinke, S.P., Blythe, B.J., & Barth, R.P. (1982). Child maltreatment and mentally retarded parents: Is there a relationship? *Mental Retardation, 20,* 201-209.

Seagull, E.A.W. & Scheurer, S.L. (1986). Neglected and abused children of mentally retarded parents. *Child Abuse and Neglect, 10,* 493-500.

Shaw, C.H. & Wright, C.H. (1960). The married mental defective. *The Lancet,* January 13, 273-274.

Tymchuk, A. & Andron, L. (1990). Mothers with mental retardation who do not abuse or neglect their children. *Child Abuse and Neglect, 14,* 313-323.

Weikert, D.P., Hohmann, M., & Banet, B. (1979). *The cognitively oriented curriculum.* Ypsilanti, MI: High Scope Educational Foundation.

Whitman, B.Y. & Accardo, P.J. (1990). Epidemiological probes: Agency surveys and Needs assessment questionnaires. In B.Y. Whitman & P.J. Accardo (Eds.), *When a parent is mentally retarded.* Baltimore: Paul H. Brookes Publishing Co.

Whitman, B.Y., Accardo, P.J., Boyert, M.M., Kendagor, R. (1990). Homelessness and cognitive performance in children: A possible link. *Social Work, 35,* 516-519.

Whitman, B.Y., Graves, B., & Accardo, P.J. (1987). The mentally retarded parent in the community: Identification method and needs assessment survey. *American Journal of Mental Deficiency, 91,* 636-638.

Whitman, B., Graves, B., & Accardo, P.J. (1990). Parents Learning Together I. In B.Y. Whitman & P.J. Accardo (Eds.), *When a parent is mentally retarded.* Baltimore: Paul H. Brookes Publishing Co.

Sexual Assault
and People with Disabilities

Arlene Bowers Andrews
Lois J. Veronen

SUMMARY. After years of neglect, societal concern has begun to focus on sexual assault and people with disabilities. The prevalence of sexual victimization is at least as common for people with disabilities as for other people, perhaps more common, particularly for acquaintance rape. This review examines relevant factors, including vulnerability, impact of sexual victimization, assistance needs, and recovery. Individual service plans should always include risk assessments and security plans to promote risk reduction.

The recent rise in societal concern for the rights and needs of people with disabilities coincides with increasing concern for victim rights and needs. Substantial information has evolved regarding the devastating physical, material, and psychosocial costs of victimization. Research has established that of the many types of victimization, sexual assault is likely to produce the worst psychosocial impacts (Kilpatrick, Saunders, Amick-McMullan, Best, Veronen, & Resnick, 1989; Kilpatrick, Saunders, Veronen, Best & Von, 1987).

Despite these advances, knowledge about sexual assault and people with disabilities is still sparse. Methodological challenges and attitudinal barriers have deterred empirical studies. For example, typical victimization prevalence and incidence studies use telephone interviews with randomly sampled households from the general population. Such studies fail to reach people with mental disabilities and communication disorders and people who live in institutions. Additionally, the 1980s Zeitgeist in the field of disabilities focused on goals of independence, integration, and productivity. Research suggesting negative aspects to those goals, such as a possible increase in victimization, would have been perceived as contrary to prevailing values and would be unlikely to generate support. The 1990s Zeitgeist has become more moderate, focused on inclusion, interdependence, contribution, and acknowledgement of risks that confront all people, regardless of ability level.

PROBLEM OVERVIEW

Understanding the implications of sexual assault for people with disabilities begins with basic definitions, typical dynamics, prevalence indicators, special attention to matters of acquaintance rape and informed consent, and information about perpetrators with disabilities.

Basic Definitions

For purposes of this article, *disability* is defined as "a physical or mental impairment that substantially limits one or more of the major life activities" of an individual (Americans with Disabilities Act, 42 United States Code, Sec. 12102). This definition applies to persons of any age and is more inclusive than the developmental disabilities definition which requires impairment in three or more areas (Developmental Disabilities Assistance and Bill of Rights Act of 1984, P.L. 98-527).

Definitions of sexual assault vary widely. Here, *sexual assault* is defined as any unwanted sexual activity or sexual activity that is obtained without consent. The latter includes situations in which people with mental disabilities that limit their capacity to give consent are enticed into sexual activity. Sexual assault includes rape, exhibitionism, and pornographic situations, such as when a person is required to view or listen to objectionable material or be photographed as a subject. Sexual assault may be verbal in the form of phone calls, letters, or direct communication. *Rape* and attempted rape are situations in which sexual contact has been obtained by force or threat of force.

Typical Dynamics of Sexual Assault

Some of the more traumatic assaults are sudden, involving brutal force. Others are more subtle and manipulative. Sex offenders often overcome verbal and physical resistance by seductively offering attention, affection, rewards, and bribes in exchange for sexual contact. They usually back these with threats of physical or emotional harm, such as humiliation, loss of residential security, or family disruption if the victim tells someone about the assaults (Groth, 1979).

Sexual assault is an act of violence, a pervasive intrusion. In rape, the victim is forced to take another person into his or her body. In other assaults, the victim may be touched, fondled, have contact with the perpetrator's sexual organs, or be forced to perform acts against his or her will. Sexual assault survivors frequently feel overwhelmed, helpless, and afraid that death is imminent. Even when the assault involves no contact or force, survivors often feel violated, through body, mind, spirit, and emotions.

The occurrence of an act of sexual assault depends on many factors (Andrews, 1992; Russell, 1984). The perpetrator must have the predisposition as well as the motivation and the ability to perform the act. Perpetrators are propelled to aggression because of needs or motives and the inadequacy of intrapersonal or external restraints. Whether an assault actually occurs or not depends on situational factors which increase the opportunity for it to occur. These situational risk factors include the victim's condition and behavior, the physical environment (for example: isolated, dark) and the social environment (for example: unsupervised, use of alcohol or other drugs, inadequate social support). A person is at risk of sexual victimization when in the presence of a potential perpetrator in a nonsecure situation. Most perpetrators are relatives or acquaintances of the victims.

Incidence and Prevalence

Rape and sexual assault are tragically common. Between 20% and 30% of women and 10% of men in the U.S. will experience at least one rape or rape attempt (Ellis, 1989; Finkelhor, 1979). As many as 40% of men and 1% of women are at risk of committing forced sexual activity (Ellis, 1989). People are at risk of sexual assault throughout their lifetimes, from soon after birth through very old age. The authors are aware of victims as young as 3 weeks and as old as 78 years.

Nobody seems to keep appropriate statistics to estimate incidence or prevalence of sexual assault against people with disabilities. Agencies that serve people with disabilities omit victimization from routine recording, and are unlikely to have workers skilled at detecting less obvious forms of victimization. Agencies that serve victims omit identification of disabilities from their records and are unlikely to have workers skilled at detecting less obvious disabilities. Although no national prevalence studies have been conducted regarding sexual assault and people with disabilities, anecdotal records and the reports of professionals who work with disabilities and/or sexual assault suggest the sexual victimization rates are high.

In one study of persons with congenital physical disabilities, 8 of 26 (31%) reported sexual abuse histories (Brown, 1988). In a sample of 87 adolescent girls with mental retardation, 22 (25%) were sexually abused (Chamberlain, Rauh, Passer, McGrath, & Burket, 1984). Of 150 multihandicapped children aged 3 to 19 admitted to a psychiatric hospital, 36% had histories of sexual abuse (Ammerman, Van Hasselt, Hersen, McGonigle, & Lubetsky, 1989). Over 50% of women who were blind from birth reported one or more forced sexual experiences (Welbourne, Lipschitz, Selvin, & Green, 1983). Many clinicians believe hard-of-hearing women are at greater risk of sexual assault than others (Cowgell, 1980).

When reports by victim services specialists are considered, indicators emerge which suggest people with disabilities are over-represented in their services populations. In Boston, 2%-15% of sexual assault services recipients had physical, psychiatric, or sensory disabilities (Moglia, 1986). Given that few victim services specialists are trained to identify, assess, or serve individuals with disabilities, these figures are likely to be severe underestimates.

The available information suggests victims with disabilities are most likely to be assaulted by someone they know. In Seattle, the perpetrator was a relative or caretaker in 99% of rape cases involving victims with disabilities (Cole, 1986). As persons with disabilities are integrated or included into more diverse living and employment situations, their risk of assault by strangers may increase as exposure to a wider range of persons, including potential perpetrators, increases.

Women are at particular risk for sexual assault throughout their lives. The annual incidence of reported sexual assault against women over age 50 is 2-19 per 1,000 (Davis & Brody, 1979). As people get older, they are more likely to acquire disabilities. The rate of sexual assault is less frequent than for younger groups, but the physical, financial, and psychosocial costs are perceived as more severe by older survivors (Steinmetz, 1988; U.S. House of Representatives Select Committee on Aging, 1990). Sexual assault may induce a disability at any age, but especially during old age. The case of Ms. M, a 78-year-old woman, illustrates the devastating effect of sexual assault in old age. She lived alone, carried out a busy social life, and played bridge twice a week. Within six months following a brutal rape in her own home, her overall physical and psychological condition deteriorated dramatically. She suffered severe cognitive deterioration and depression. She could no longer live alone or care for herself, so her family decided to move her to a nursing home.

Obviously, many people with physical and mental disabilities suffer sexual victimization. Their numbers are apparently high, although precisely undetermined. Research is needed to better establish incidence and prevalence rates.

Acquaintance Rape and Matters of Informed Consent

Acquaintance rape ("date rape") may be the most common form of sexual assault. In a nationally representative sample of 3,187 college women and 2,972 college men, Koss (1988) found that 15.4% of the women reported experiencing and 4.4% of the men reported perpetrating, since age 14, an act that could be legally considered rape. An additional 12.1% of the women experienced attempted rape, and 11.9% of the women experienced coerced sex that was not legally rape. Another study found that 15% of a sample of college men reported obtaining sexual intercourse against their date's will (Rapaport & Burkhart, 1984).

Many acquaintance rape victims fail to realize they have been raped. They may have entered a situation with an acquaintance expecting to have an affectionate exchange with no or limited sexual contact. They may have felt ambivalent about their relationships and unsure of how to respond as the pressure for sex from their partners escalated. They objected, perhaps vehemently, but were sexually used anyway. The perpetrators ignored the objections, perhaps sensing the victims' interest in friendly relationships, and mistakenly interpreting this as ambivalence over the desire to have sex.

Even more people have experienced unwanted sexual advances, such as fondling and harassment, that are less intrusive than rape. People with disabilities whose social and sexual education has been restricted or neglected may be at particular risk for these forms of assault. Considerable social skill is required to repel exploitive sexual behavior in its early stages, before it advances into aggression. Without appropriate and specific training in handling such approaches, the victim may feel extreme discomfort, guilt, and powerlessness if the offender begins to advance.

Informed consent is the foundation of a healthy sexual relationship (Ames, Hepner, Kaeser, & Penler, 1988). The issue of consent is easier to conceptualize for the person who has no disabilities that interfere with his or her capacity to communicate or reason. The unchallenged person may be able to discuss feelings, wants, and desires. For people with mental disabilities and communication disorders, consent issues become more complex. They have a right to consensual sex, but must be protected from nonconsensual harm and exploitation.

The issue of sexuality for persons with disabilities and how to determine when consent can be given is receiving increasing attention from professionals, particularly since legal rights to consensual sexual expression are becoming more clearly determined. The American Association for the Mentally Retarded has a special interest group of professionals involved with sexuality issues. It currently appears that the trend among programs serving clients with mental disabilities is to make individual determinations for each client, using specific criteria. An example of criteria is found in a legal analysis for balancing the individual rights of sexual expression and state duty to protect from harm, prepared by the New York Commission on the Quality of Care (Stavis & Bishop, 1991). According to the legal analysis, three elements are essential for consent: (1) knowledge by the individual of the nature of the activity; (2) intelligence of the individual in realizing the benefits and risk of the activity and a demonstrated ability to rationally process the knowledge and apply it to personal standards of living; and (3) voluntariness or a free decision to choose to engage in or refrain from sexual activity. If this model is widely adopted, programs for persons with dependency needs will be expected to conduct educational activities regarding sexuality and the consequences of sexual behavior and to assess client voluntariness, probably through an interdisciplinary team.

The Perpetrator with a Disability

Information about disabilities among perpetrators is even more sparse than information about victims with disabilities. One can assume that the sexually aggressive population includes people with disabilities and that they require treatment suited to their needs.

The few available studies tend to focus on perpetrators with mental or intellectual impairment. For example, about half of female sex offenders have mental illness, mental retardation, brain damage, or psychosis (Grayson, 1989). Considerable attention has been given to the false notion, fueled by historic prejudice, that people with mental retardation commonly commit sexual offenses. In fact the rates of sexual offenses for populations with mental retardation appear to be no different than other populations and may be lower (Schilling & Schinke, 1989). However, the offender with mental retardation is less likely than an offender with higher intelligence level to devise schemes to avoid apprehension, and thus is more likely to get caught.

People with intellectual impairments may be at risk of being charged with sexual offenses for reasons of naivete rather than the more typical motives of anger and/or the desire for power (Groth, 1979). Through social learning the typical sex offender develops sexual preferences for specific activities such as child molestation, overpowering acquaintances, or ritualistic use of force. People with intellectual impairments may end up in sexually aggressive situations for different reasons. Their social isolation and inadequate education about sexuality may hinder their accurate interpretation of social cues, including resistance messages from the victim. Survivors of untreated sexual exploitation may pass on learned inappropriate sexual behavior, especially in acquaintance situations with peers who similarly have limited intellectual functioning. Solid education about sexuality and interpersonal skills can help to prevent such situations. Similarly, parents with intellectual impairment have been known to unwittingly enable their children to enter into sexually exploitive relationships. These parents need special training and support to enhance their protective responsibilities to their children.

Some sex offenders who are motivated by anger and power also have disabilities. Sex offender treatment programs should be adapted to meet their special needs. Many treatment models are used with offenders. Most generally teach offenders to examine and accept responsibility for their behavior and learn prosocial methods of sexual and emotional gratification. Swanson and Garwick (1990) describe a program which holds the sex offender accountable while providing a realistic appraisal of intellectual strengths and weaknesses, training in sexual and social skills, and coordination of specialists to treat related problems (e.g., substance abuse, adaptation to impairment).

VULNERABILITY TO VICTIMIZATION

People with disabilities may be more likely than other people to be sexually assaulted. Professionals widely accept this based on their practice experience, even though little empirical research has been conducted to confirm this informed belief.

Many factors influence the risk for sexual assault and neglect of survivor needs among people with disabilities (Aiello, 1986; Krents, Schulman, & Brenner, 1987; Longo & Gochenour, 1981; Moglia, 1986; Musick, 1984; Rinear, 1985; Schor, 1987; Stuart & Stuart, 1981; Tharinger, Horton, & Millea, 1990; Worthington, 1984). A review of the literature and the authors' experience with survivors reveals eight factors associated with vulnerability to victimization among persons with disabilities.

1. People with severe disabilities may be dependent on others for long-term care, leading them to be compliant and trusting of caregivers, including those who assault or exploit them. Those who are dependent on others for personal care such as toileting or bathing are particularly vulnerable to situations that may be sexually confusing or exploitive. Dependence may hinder their willingness to disclose or seek help, as in a case reported by Moglia (1986). A girl with cerebral palsy, sexually assaulted by her stepfather and forced into prostitution by both parents, said she was afraid to tell anyone because she believed the parents would stop caring for her. On another extreme, children raised in highly protective homes are at risk of failing to learn adequate self-protective skills, so that when they become more independent, they inadequately detect danger.

People with disabilities who live in institutions (including convalescent and nursing homes, community boarding homes, and psychiatric and mental retardation facilities) are at exceptional risk. Their disabilities may be more severe, and fewer situational safeguards exist to protect them from potential harm. When the sex offender is on staff, he/she may control the resident's situation through bribes such as grounds privileges and furloughs or threats such as seclusion, restriction, and delayed release. Musick (1984) found that many institutional sexual assaults occurred while patients were helpless, heavily medicated, comatose, or in restraints.

2. People with disabilities are still denied basic human rights. Even though laws have changed, personal and institutional practices improve more slowly. As victims of historical oppression and negative social attitudes and behaviors, people with disabilities may feel more powerless than other people. They are vulnerable to exploitation by assailants whom they perceive as powerful, who can induce even greater harm or deny basic life supports if they fail to cooperate. They may require special support to believe in their own power and ability to resist assault. Their support systems may be inadequate or unprepared to deal with sexual victimization. They may hesitate to ask for help because they mistrust the competence of care providers to respond to their particular needs as survivors with disabilities (a correct assumption, based on information discussed earlier).

Denying human rights of a person with a disability and negative attitudes toward a rape victim are illustrated in the case of Ms. G. She is a kind, gentle woman with mild mental retardation who is now in her early 50s. She was the youngest by seven years in a family of three children. Her retardation resulted from prolonged labor and oxygen deprivation during birth. Her family was upper-middle class, conservative, and very religious. As a girl of 15, Ms. G was raped by a group of older boys from her school. However, during the 1950s this event was not considered a rape. One of the boys, whom Ms. G considered a friend, had convinced her to go to an abandoned building, where she expected to see a kitten or puppy. Three other boys were waiting there. The boys began to kiss her, touch her breasts and genitals, and take off her clothes. She began to cry and asked them to stop, but they continued. Each of the boys had intercourse with her. Ms. G arrived home, confused and upset, two hours later than expected. She tearfully told her mother. Her father was angry at her for going off with one of the boys, an act he regarded as poor judgement and uncontrollable "boy craziness." She was not treated as a victim. Instead, she was punished, taken to a physician, and sterilized. Her parents believed her presumed interest in boys would decrease and they would no longer need to be concerned about her sexual behavior. Ms. G never dated and never married; she has spent her life caring for other people's children.

3. Offenders may target people with disabilities because they believe there is less risk of discovery. Offenders, driven by anger and the desire for power, devalue victims in general. They may assume a hearing impairment means the victim cannot call for help, a visual impairment precludes the victim aiding in detection, or that the person with mental retardation cannot understand.

Two case situations illustrate this vulnerability. These cases occurred in different employment settings, but the dynamics are similar. Men in supervisory positions ("the bosses") took women with mild retardation off the job, initially telling them they had some special work for them to do. Once away from the job site, the men coerced the women into having intercourse or performing sexual acts. Initially neither woman told anyone. After repeated incidents, each told someone in her personal network. The management of the companies were informed and the assaults ceased. However, the lack of evidence and apparent lack of resistance by the victims led local prosecutors to refuse to prosecute the cases.

4. Many survivors encounter difficulty in being believed. People with disabilities have to deal with additional resistance from potential helpers due to prevalent false beliefs that people with disabilities are immune from assault because they are asexual, pitied, or undesirable. Professionals may fail to report suspected cases to authorities and may not refer survivors for recovery assistance because of such biases.

People with mental disabilities encounter exceptional resistance to the credibility of their assault reports. Staff at psychiatric hospitals, for example, may interpret a patient's report as a fabricated symptom of the illness, or as a distortion of a consensual sexual relationship. Raped psychiatric patients have been described as "sexually acting out" (Musick, 1984). Persons with mental retardation encounter similar difficulty, given false staff perceptions that they are sexually driven and "ask for it."

5. People with intellectual impairments are less likely to have been educated about sexuality, so they may be less able to recognize, understand, and resist sexually abusive or exploitive situations. They may doubt their perceptions when they are in suspicious situations. They may be unskilled at handling sexual advances, as noted in the section on acquaintance rape.

6. People with disabilities may be relatively socially isolated and lonely, more vulnerable to exploitation through manipulative relationships that initially appear to be affectionate and indicative of social acceptance. Their emotional and social needs may lead them to be easily led, wanting to please their associates.

The case of Margaret illustrates this issue. Margaret was a 16-year-old female with mental retardation who stayed at home all day throughout summer vacation. She was very lonely and had few friends or social contacts other than her family. Margaret's brother-in-law began to show her special attention. He worked as a yard man, with irregular hours. He began to visit in the middle of the day. Initially, he was nice, but then he began to pressure her to have sex with him. She wanted to please him and eventually gave in. The relationship was discovered only after she became pregnant.

7. People with disabilities may be more challenged in attempts to

take risk-reducing precautions or to resist actual assaults (Davis & Brody, 1979). Because of challenges posed by disability, they may rely upon set routines, easily observable by potential assailants. They may be dependent on public transportation, sometimes accessible only at vulnerable locations. People with sensory and perceptual disabilities may be unable to detect approaching danger. If attacked, the struggle with an assailant may be ineffective, perhaps due to lack of physical strength or experience in resisting. All victims feel helpless, but persons with disabilities may feel helpless to an even greater extent.

8. The values and attitudes within the field of disabilities toward mainstreaming and integration without consideration for each individual's capacity for self-protection may place persons at higher risk for victimization (Veronen & Robinson, 1990). The full integration of persons with disabilities into work situations often means the person with mental retardation is working in a semi-skilled or unskilled position, at or below minimum wage, during evening or night hours or split shifts. Co-workers are frequently persons with drug, alcohol, or untreated emotional problems. Group homes are often in high-crime neighborhoods. Persons with disabilities must travel through risky means, such as public buses, taxis, or paying coworkers for rides.

These eight factors increase vulnerability and suggest that people with disabilities are at considerable risk for sexual victimization. Even so, alarmingly little attention tends to be given to their needs for security, protection, and specialized help when victimized.

CHALLENGES CONFRONTING PEOPLE WITH DISABILITIES WHO ARE SEXUALLY VICTIMIZED

Sexual assault survivors with disabilities may be challenged by the impact of the victimization, the process of disclosure and reporting, and the search for assistance and recovery support.

Impact of the Victimization

When assaulted, people with disabilities may be more vulnerable to serious or lasting damage than people without disabilities (Camblin, 1982; Tharinger et al., 1990). Sexual assault can induce physical, psychological, social, and financial harm for any survivor. How an individual responds to an assault or an exploitive relationship depends on a number of factors, including but not limited to the individual's psychosocial functioning prior to the assault, the nature of the assault (e.g., intensity, duration, intrusiveness), the role of the survivor during the assault, relationship to the perpetrator, and the context of post-assault support. All survivors are likely to feel alone, to experience self-blame, and low self-esteem. Survivors with disabilities may feel these responses are due to their disabilities; they may be unaware that these are typical survivor responses.

Physical and mental disabilities may be exacerbated by sexual assault. Specific physical disabilities pose unique challenges to survivors and their care providers (Stuart, 1986; Stuart & Stuart, 1981). A series of examples follows.

All survivors are likely to feel isolated, but people with hearing impairments may feel particularly lonely; the severely impaired will need interpreters. Disorientation is a common response of all survivors and may be extreme among those who have visual impairment. Caregivers should take time to help the victim feel grounded. Trauma can magnify speech problems, so a person listening to a survivor with speech impairment must be particularly patient, clearly asking questions of the victim, respectfully asking for repetition if answers are indistinct. Survivors with mobility impairments may require special transportation throughout emergency intervention and recovery.

Of course all survivor service facilities should be wheelchair-accessible. All survivors tend to feel powerless and should be treated in ways to help them regain a sense of personal power. A survivor with spinal-cord injury should be asked about preferred method if he or she needs to be moved or examined. Diabetic survivors may develop insulin shock following the trauma of assault. Their symptoms or those of survivors with cerebral palsy can be mistaken by untrained persons as signs of intoxication (slurred speech, unsteady gait, disorientation, confusion). Careful screening and medical attention is critical.

Similarly, people with mental disabilities require appropriate care. When a survivor is intellectually impaired, therapists, law

enforcement investigators, and recovery workers need to accommodate her or his special communication and education needs. People
with mental retardation may be confused and may need to unlearn
inappropriate behaviors acquired through sexual victimization. All
survivors struggle for cognitive understanding of their victimization
and may have difficulty organizing their thoughts or concentrating.
Survivors with learning disabilities are particularly challenged by
this effect.

People with emotional and psychiatric disabilities probably have
the worst problems in being believed. Many people have the attitude that people with emotional or mental illness are fabricating
sexual assault stories because of their illnesses. The psychosocial
damage induced by sexual assault is extensive for any survivor.
People with pre-existing emotional and psychological problems are
likely to demonstrate more serious mental health problems after
assault (Figley, 1985; 1986). For example, a study of 87 sexually
abused children with emotional disabilities demonstrates the variety
of emotional damage that can occur (Garbarino, Brookhouser, &
Authier, 1987). Those who externalized their disturbance showed
poor peer relationships, seductive and/or promiscuous behavior,
running away, substance abuse, and aggression. Those who inter-
nalized exhibited excessive compliance, extraordinary fears, depression, regressive behavior, and suicidal ideation.

Each survivor of sexual assault is unique, requiring specialized
attention. When the survivor has a disability, it can be identified and
accommodated as part of a comprehensive response to individual
needs.

Disclosure and Reporting

Official reporting rates to protective service and law enforcement
agencies are one indicator of whether a survivor is receiving help or
not. Most people who are sexually assaulted fail to report it to
authorities; people with disabilities are even less likely to report
(Aiello, 1986; Brown, 1988; Krents, Schulman, & Brenner, 1987;
Tharinger et al., 1990). Many survivors encounter disbelief when
they try to report; survivors with disabilities may encounter particular resistance stemming from untrained officials' false stereotypes

about disabilities and sexuality. If a survivor does not make an official report, he or she may disclose the sexual abuse to a trusted friend or family member. Unfortunately, some survivors cannot or do not tell anyone.

Survivors with disabilities may be unable or hesitant to disclose for many reasons. They tend to be relatively socially isolated, and may be uninformed about where to turn for help. Communication difficulties may deter them, or they may fear others will fail to believe them. Some may fear retaliation by the perpetrator. Sexual assault survivors often feel guilty, confused, and responsible; survivors with disabilities, like other survivors, may blame themselves. In cases of acquaintance rape, they may tolerate the victimization in order to feel more accepted or like other people.

People with severe disabilities may be unable to communicate. In at least one case, a man had sexual relations with his wife who was in a coma. Since the couple lived in a state with no marital rape law, no charges could be brought against him. In another case, a woman became pregnant while in a coma, hospitalized. The perpetrator was never detected.

The first step toward victim assistance is disclosure or reporting. All people need education about how to detect high risk situations and how to get help when victimized. Caregivers must create supportive environments for people who need assistance in disclosing their experiences.

Survivor Assistance and Recovery

Like all sexual assault survivors, those with disabilities need compassionate and individually appropriate care. Skilled physical and psychological first aid are essential during the immediate aftermath of an assault or the disclosure of a past assault. The medical examination can be particularly traumatic because it is conducted not only for the victim's well-being but also to gather legal evidence. The weeks following an assault can be devastating as the survivor traverses legal, medical, and psychosocial services systems and deals with relatives, friends, and colleagues. Sexual assault crisis and support centers exist across the nation to help survivors cope, survive the traumatic response, and move toward stability and recovery. Effective services programs will accommodate the needs of survivors with any type disability through assessment procedures, trained caregivers, barrier-free services, and special protective interventions.

1. *Assessment.* Burgess and Holmstrom (1978) recommend several steps for survivor service providers to follow in assessing and responding to the needs of sexual assault survivors with disabilities. All providers should be trained to suspect the presence of disabilities and either identify or seek skilled assistance in determining the presence of a disability. The provider should determine if the disability will affect the interview and helping process. The survivor should first be asked; then, if necessary, help should be obtained from someone who is familiar with such disability (family member, friend, staff member, designated consultant or volunteer). The survivor services provider should proceed with the regular protocol, making appropriate adaptations as necessary. When a survivor is already involved with other agencies, representatives of those agencies may be contacted, if the survivor gives permission. Careful assessment procedures will increase detection and the likelihood that the survivor's needs will be appropriately met.

2. *Trained caregivers.* Survivor services providers, including law enforcement personnel, prosecutors, lawyers, judges, health, and psychosocial caregivers, need to be trained in how to recognize and effectively respond to disabilities (Aiello, Capkin, & Catania, 1983). Likewise, people who are specialists in the care of persons with disabilities need training regarding recognition and response to sexual trauma. Agencies that specialize in disabilities services may designate one or more personnel to serve as in-house victimization specialists. The specialists could serve as resource persons to staff and survivors, providing such services as education about risk reduction, crisis support and recovery assistance for survivors, and training for staff in how to assess client victimization history. Skilled collaboration among specialists in both fields–victim services and disability services–is critical for effective care of the survivor with a disability.

3. *Barrier-free services.* Every victim-serving agency should have a strong commitment to nondiscrimination and inclusion (Aiello & Capkin, 1984). Additionally, agencies can actively reach

out to assure availability of care to persons with disabilities. Examples of actions to eliminate barriers to care include (a) public awareness activities that target people with disabilities; (b) information and referral services that screen for callers with disabilities and provide access to those with speech and hearing impairments; (c) 24-hour availability of appropriate transportation, interpreters, communication assistance, and public transportation for emergency intervention; (d) physical accessibility of all facilities; (e) designated personnel who are trained to respond to victims with disabilities at survivor services agencies; (f) designated personnel trained to monitor risk reduction and respond to victims at agencies that serve people with disabilities; (g) adaptive services by medical practitioners, psychotherapists, and others so that special needs are met (e.g., home-based crisis and recovery counseling). Of course, every agency should work to promote an *inclusive atmosphere* where survivors with disabilities feel accepted by other clients as well as caregivers, particularly when they must reside in facilities such as emergency shelters. Such actions result in increased consciousness of and more skilled responses to survivors with disabilities.

4. *Special protective interventions.* People with disabilities are entitled to special protective interventions by state and local authorities when they have been assaulted by caregivers in their own homes or in institutions in which they reside. All states have child abuse reporting laws and most have similar laws regarding the protection of vulnerable adults, persons age 18 or older who have intellectual impairments or other challenges which interfere with their abilities to seek protection on their own. These laws mandate or encourage the reporting of all forms of suspected abuse to child or adult protection authorities, who investigate and initiate assistance to protect the victim. Advocates must be aware that people with disabilities are often overlooked because, in most areas of the U.S., the protective services systems are part of a public welfare system that is overwhelmed and in perpetual crisis.

People with disabilities who are sexually abused by persons other than their caretakers can look to rape crisis and support networks and law enforcement agencies for assistance. Many states have crime victim/witness assistance programs, often located in prosecutor's offices, law enforcement agencies, or independent agencies.

Advocates must work to assure these programs respond appropriately to survivors with disabilities.

PREVENTION AND RISK REDUCTION

Sexual assault prevention programs have two general foci: (a) individuals, to reduce the likelihood that they will become victims or perpetrators, and (b) social and physical environments, to increase their security.

All people need skills to reduce the risk that victimization will occur and resist severe damage when an attack does occur. They can be prepared for psychological and physical defensive action during an attack, to reduce the severity of harm, and they can understand how to get help if an attack occurs. None of these actions places responsibility on the victim for preventing an assault—only the perpetrator can truly prevent the act. The victim is never to blame when an assault occurs. Knowledgeable anticipation can help people feel less fearful and more empowered regarding how to cope with the risks of being assaulted.

Risk reduction generally involves training people to practice avoidance behaviors, physical design measures, and community organization. Avoidance behaviors include such actions as always making a living unit look occupied; arranging for someone to make daily telephone contact; never opening a door to a stranger without ascertaining identification; travelling with a companion when possible; or staying inside a dysfunctional car. Numerous materials and training programs are available to help people learn to avoid risky situations (Benedict, 1987; Castleman, 1984; Davis & Brody, 1979; Duncan, 1980; National Crime Prevention Institute, 1986; O'Day, Specktor, Sayles, Bauman, & Exley, 1983; Stock, 1975). Some suggestions aim to deter an attack, others advise what to do when under attack. Verbal and physical self-defense classes can be adapted for people with specific disabilities.

Physical design measures include such arrangements as adequate locks on doors, alarm systems, fencing, and lighting. Community organization includes such actions as knowing one's neighbors and participating in Neighborhood Watch activities. Most of these activities are designed to increase surveillance over a physical area to deter potential perpetrators and sound alerts when suspicious activities occur.

Any person with a disability who is developing a plan for independent living should be entitled to a risk assessment, facilitated by trained professionals, and a plan for security and protection. The plan could include such elements as changes in the physical environment, individualized education regarding precautionary behaviors, and procedures for mobilization of protective resources when necessary. A resource person could be designated for the person to contact when a sexually confusing or suspicious event occurs.

Institutions that provide residential care for people with disabilities can develop internal procedures to reduce the risk of sexual assault. Such action includes educating all staff regarding sexual assault, enforcing policies and laws regarding mistreatment of residents, submitting to regular external institutional reviews regarding resident safety, screening all employees for sexual abuse histories, and increasing security procedures, including the surveillance of isolated areas. Every institution should have a victimization risk reduction plan to promote the safety of its residents. Advocates for people with disabilities should routinely assess the security of institutional environments and insist upon organizational security and protection plans that specifically address sexual victimization.

To minimize the risk that people will become sex offenders, prosocial skills education and solid social supports starting in early childhood are essential. Developmentally appropriate education about sexuality and interpersonal relations is particularly critical for young people with intellectual disabilities, to reduce the possibility that naive assaults will occur. Identification and psychosocial treatment of childhood abuse and other traumas can diminish the risks of antisocial reactions, including sexually assaultive behavior.

Primary prevention of sexual assault against people with disabilities is founded in eliminating negative stereotypes and false beliefs, particularly regarding their sexuality, rights, and power. Mass education of the public is the means to address this problem. Additionally, as social competence of people with disabilities is promoted and supported, their vulnerability to assault will be reduced.

CONCLUSION

People with disabilities are challenged by sexual victimization risks and needs. Once considered invulnerable to sexual victimization or inconsequential among survivor populations, the person with a disability has become recognized as someone vulnerable to sexual assault, able to reduce risks, and entitled to appropriate assistance when assault happens.

Practitioners in the specialty fields of victim services and services to people with disabilities have considerable work to do to assure widespread policies and programs for the prevention and treatment of sexual assault against persons with disabilities. The vulnerability factors require focused attention. Many people with disabilities are dependent on caregivers, perceived as powerless, and exceptionally devalued by perpetrators. Some are sexually naive and socially isolated, at particular risk of sexual exploitation by caregivers and acquaintances. The cultural denial of their sexuality imposes barriers when they seek help for sexual victimization. Change efforts need to focus on strengthening the risk resistance of people with disabilities, enlightening and enabling caregivers to effectively respond to the sexual concerns of people with disabilities, and promoting societal norms and attitudes that convey respect for bodily integrity and affirmation of the right to protection.

REFERENCES

Aiello, D. (1986). Issues and concerns confronting disabled assault victims: Strategies for treatment and prevention. *Sexuality and Disability, 7*(3-4), 96-101.

Aiello, D. & Capkin, L. (1984). Services for disabled victims: Elements and standards. *Response*, Fall, 14-16.

Aiello, D., Capkin, L., & Catania, H. (1983). Strategies and techniques for serving the disabled assault victim: A pilot training program for providers and consumers. *Sexuality and Disability, 6* (3/4), 135-144.

Americans with Disabilities Act, 42 United States Code, Sec. 12102.

Ames, T.H., Hepner, P.J., Kaeser, F., & Penler, B. (1988). *Guidelines for sexuality education and programming for the next decade*. As quoted in D. Tharinger, C.B. Horton, & S. Millea (1990), Sexual abuse and exploitation of children and adults with mental retardation and other handicaps, *Child Abuse and Neglect, 14*, 304.

Ammerman, R.T., Van Hasselt, V.B., Hersen, M., McGonigle, J.J., & Lubetsky,

M.J. (1989). Abuse and neglect in psychiatrically hospitalized multihandi-capped children, *Child Abuse and Neglect, 13*, 335-343.

Andrews, A.B. (1992). *Victimization and survivor services.* NY: Springer-Verlag New York Inc.

Benedict, H. (1987). *Safe, strong, and streetwise.* Boston: Little, Brown & Co.

Brown, D.E. (1988). Factors affecting psychosexual development of adults with congenital physical disabilities. *Physical and Occupational Therapy in Pediatrics, 8*(2/3), 43-58.

Burgess, A.W. & Holmstrom, L.L. (1978). Complicating factors in rape: Adolescent case illustrations. In A.W. Burgess, A.N. Groth, L.L. Holmstrom, & S.M. Sgroi (Eds.), *Sexual assault of children and adolescents,* Lexington, Mass.: Lexington Books, 61-83.

Camblin, L.D. (1982). A survey of state efforts in gathering information on child abuse and neglect in handicapped populations. *Child Abuse and Neglect, 6,* 465-472.

Castleman, M. (1984). *Crime free.* NY: Simon & Schuster Inc.

Chamberlain, A., Rauh, J., Passer, A., McGrath, M., & Burket, R. (1984). Issues in fertility control for mentally retarded female adolescents I: Sexual activity, sexual abuse, and contraception. *Pediatrics, 73,* 445-450.

Cole, S.S. (1986). Facing the challenges of sexual abuse in persons with disabilities. *Sexuality and Disability, 7*(3-4), 71-88.

Cowgell, V.G. (1980). Criminal victimization of the hearing-impaired: A research paper. Available from Counseling and Placement Center, Gallaudet University, Washington, DC 20002.

Davis, L.J. & Brody, E.M. (1979). *Rape and older women: A guide to prevention and protection.* Rockville, MD: National Institute of Mental Health.

Developmental Disabilities Assistance and Bill of Rights Act of 1984, P.L. 98-527.

Duncan, J.T.S. (1980). *Citizen crime prevention tactics: A literature review and selected bibliography.* Washington, DC: U.S. Dept. of Justice, NCJ 65156.

Ellis, L. (1989). *Theories of rape: Inquiries into the causes of sexual aggression.* NY: Hemisphere Publishing.

Figley, C.R. (Ed.) (1985). *Trauma and its wake: Vol. I.* NY: Brunner/Mazel, Inc.

Figley, C.R. (Ed.) (1986). *Trauma and its wake: Vol. II.* NY: Brunner/Mazel, Inc.

Finkelhor, D. (1979). *Sexually victimized children.* NY: The Free Press.

Garbarino, J., Brookhouser, P.E., & Authier, K.J. (1987). *Special children, special risks: The maltreatment of children with disabilities.* NY: Aldine de Gruyter.

Grayson, J. (1989). Female sex offenders. *Virginia Child Protection Newsletter, 28,* 1, 5-8, 12-13.

Groth, A.N. (1979). *Men who rape: The psychology of the offender.* NY: Plenum Publishing Corp.

Kilpatrick, D.G., Saunders, B.E., Amick-McMullan, A., Best, C.L., Veronen, L.J., & Resnick, H. (1989). Factors affecting the development of crime-related post-traumatic stress disorder. *Behavior Therapy, 20,* 199-214.

Kilpatrick, D.G., Saunders, B.E., Veronen, L.J., Best, C.L., & Von, J.M. (1987).

Criminal victimization: Lifetime prevalence, reporting to police, and psychological impact. *Crime and Delinquency, 33*(4), 479-489.

Koss, M.P. (1988). Hidden rape: Sexual aggression and victimization in a national sample of students in higher education. In Burgess, A.W. (Ed.), *Rape and sexual assault II.*, NY: Garland Publishing, 3-25.

Krents, E., Schulman, V., & Brenner, S. (1987). Child abuse and the disabled child: Perspectives for parents. *Volta Review, 89* (5), 78-95.

Longo, R.E. & Gochenour, C. (1981). Sexual assault of handicapped individuals. *Journal of Rehabilitation, 47*(3), 24-27.

Moglia, R. (1986). Sexual abuse and disability. *SIECUS Report,* Mar, 9-10.

Musick, J.L. (1984). Patterns of institutional sexual assault. *Response to Violence in the Family and Sexual Assault,* 7(3), 1-2, 10-11.

National Crime Prevention Institute. (1986). *Understanding crime prevention.* Boston: Butterworths.

O'Day, B., Specktor, P., Sayles, S., Bauman, C., & Exley, P. (1983). *Preventing sexual abuse of persons with disabilities.* St. Paul, MN: Minnesota Department of Corrections.

Rapaport, K. & Burkhart, B.R. (1984). Personality and attitudinal characteristics of sexually coercive college males. *Journal of Abnormal Psychology, 93,* 216-221.

Rinear, E.E. (1985). Sexual assault and the handicapped victim. In A.W. Burgess (Ed.), *Rape and sexual assault: A research handbook,* New York: Garland, 139-145.

Russell, D.E.H. (1984). *Sexual exploitation: Rape, child sexual abuse, and workplace harassment.* Beverly Hills, CA: Sage Publications Inc.

Schilling, R.F. & Schinke, S.P. (1989). Mentally retarded sex offenders: Fact, fiction, and treatment. In J.S. Wodarski & D.L. Whitaker (Eds.), *Treatment of sex offenders in social work and mental health settings,* New York: The Haworth Press, Inc., 33-48.

Schor, D.P. (1987). Sex and sexual abuse in developmentally disabled adolescents. *Seminars in Adolescent Medicine.* New York: Thieme Medical Publishers, 1-7.

Stavis, P.F. & Bishop, K.M. (1991). Responding to sexual activity between clients: Legal and ethical dilemmas. Workshop materials presented at the New York Commission of Quality of Care. New York, NY, January 9 & 10, 1991.

Steinmetz, S.K. (1988). *Duty bound: Elder abuse and family care.* Newbury Park, CA: Sage Publications Inc.

Stock, F.P.P. (1975). *Personal safety and defense for women.* Minneapolis, MN: Burgess.

Stuart, C.K. (1986). Helping physically disabled victims of sexual assault. *Medical Aspects of Human Sexuality, 20* (11), 101-102.

Stuart, C.K. & Stuart, V.W. (1981). Sexual assault: Disabled perspective. *Sexuality and Disability, 4*(4), 246-253.

Swanson, C.K. & Garwick, G.B. (1990). Treatment for low-functioning sex offenders: Group therapy and interagency coordination. *Mental Retardation, 28* (3), 155-161.

Tharinger, D., Horton, C.B., Millea, S. (1990). Sexual abuse and exploitation of children and adults with mental retardation and other handicaps. *Child Abuse and Neglect, 14,* 301-312.

U.S. House of Representatives, Select Committee on Aging. (1990). Elder abuse: A decade of shame and inaction. Comm. Pub. No. 101-752. Washington, DC: U.S. Government Printing Office.

Veronen, L.J. & Robinson, C. (1990). Victimization among the developmentally disabled population: A cautious inquiry. Paper presented at the 98th Annual Convention of the American Psychological Association, Boston, MA.

Welbourne, A., Lipschitz, S., Selvin, H., & Green, R. (1983). A comparison of the sexual learning experiences of visually impaired and sighted women, *Journal of Visual Impairment and Blindness, 77,* 256-259.

Worthington, G.M. (1984). Sexual exploitation and abuse of people with disabilities. *Response, 7* (2), 7-8.

9780789000927